To the friends and lovers of our past and present
who provide us with a wealth of experience—
always the best teacher

What Brothers Think, What Sistahs Know About Sex

Also by Denene Millner and Nick Chiles

What Brothers Think, What Sistahs Know:
The Real Deal on Love and Relationships

By Denene Millner

The Sistahs' Rules: Secrets for Meeting,
Getting, and Keeping a Good Black Man

What Brothers Think, What Sistahs Know About Sex

The Real Deal on Passion, Loving, and Intimacy

Denene Millner and Nick Chiles

Quill
William Morrow
New York

Library of Congress Cataloging-in-Publication Data

Millner, Denene.
    What brothers think, what sistahs know about sex : the real deal
  on passion, loving, and intimacy / Denene Millner and Nick Chiles.
        p.   cm.
    ISBN 0-688-17107-9
    1. Sex.   2. Afro-American men—Sexual behavior.   3. Afro-American
  women—Sexual behavior.   I. Chiles, Nick.   II. Title.
  HQ21.M647   2000   99–36501
  306.7—dc21   CIP

Printed in the United States of America

First Edition

1   2   3   4   5   6   7   8   9   10

BOOK DESIGN BY RENATO STANISIC

www.williammorrow.com

Contents

❀

Acknowledgments

As always, we offer thanks to the Creator, who has surrounded us with the love and strength from which all of our blessings flow.

Denene: Thanks to my parents for keeping me blissfully ignorant but morally grounded—it kept me out of trouble and made me the person I am today. I'll love you both till dolphins fly and parrots swim the sea.

Nick: I can't say my parents kept me blissfully ignorant, but I thank them for providing me with a model of a prosperous union that let me know the kind of relationship I wanted—graceful, strong, unbreakable. Much love.

To Mari: It'll be at least two decades before we'll let you read this book, but you are the sun around which our world revolves.

To Mazi: You won't be reading this book for nearly a decade

and a half; we have love from here to infinity for the new "big brother."

To the family: Angelou, James, Jameelah, Troy, Maia, Imani, Zenzele, Miles—you make this life trip way more fun and worthwhile. We like you a whole lot.

To the godparents: We've been ordered not to publicly disclose your names, but y'all know who you are—we're so glad to be able to call you family now.

Thanks to our tough-as-nails agent, Eileen Cope, and the crew at Lowenstein Associates.

Hugs and smooches to Doris Cooper, our editor and sex guru. Spicy enough, Doris?

Thanks to Shawn "The Love Dove" Dove, friend and resident marketing genius.

Special thanks to Molly "Moll" Wald, the brains behind our website (www.celebrateblacklove.com). Check her out at Molli.net (and watch out Bill Gates!).

And, once again, thanks to the kitty cats, Jordan and Stark! (Leave that baby alone!)

Introduction

❧

It is one of our society's great ironies that the subject that inflames our commercial markets like a torch is still approached with hush-hush secrecy in our private lives. Most of us know more about the sexual proclivities of our forty-second president than we do about the sexual attitudes and fantasies of the person with whom we share a bed every night. Sex fascinates us. Scares us. Troubles us. Sex, not baseball, is the real Great American pastime.

And we get so much of our conception of a proper sexual life from the mass media that a part of us must always wonder: Am I normal? Is it sick for me to think that or want this? Am I doing this right?

In this book, our goal is to help people crash through those fears and insecurities by laying it all out on the table for discussion, argument, titillation, intrigue. We use our own lives, our own experiences, and our own friends as fodder to get this sex talk going. The questions can get pretty dicey—and the answers even dicier—but we have found that it is truly the thriving, unified, well-communicating couple who can talk frankly about sex. To explore each other's feelings on foreplay, performance anxiety, masturbation, pornography, infidelity, and a host of other controversial topics can be scary and thrilling at the same time. But if readers manage to work up the nerve to delve into this stuff with their paramours, we guarantee that their relationship—and especially their sex life—will advance to a better, healthier place.

Isn't it curious how much uncertainty we still carry around with us about our sex lives? We may move into an easy, comfortable communion with our partners, but how many of us are daring enough to shake things up, to bring home a bag of sex toys or a porno movie, to put on a costume and act out some of our secret sexual fantasies? In the backs of our minds, we're always wondering what our partner will think if we change up the program, introduce something drastically new. But that whole world of stimulation will suddenly be accessible if we throw open all those hidden doors for exploration.

Sex educators say it is ignorance and fear of communication that often leads our young people into ill-advised sexual behaviors such as premature, unprotected intercourse. They are afraid and ill-equipped to talk about their fears, their wishes, their limits. So instead of exploring all the ways they could pleasure each other without having sex, they go straight to the one thing they do know how to do: intercourse.

But this fear of talking about sex never really goes away completely, does it? We may become more adept at sliding into those superficial topics that we use to titillate each other, like favorite sexual positions, but most of us aren't as comfortable with deeper stuff, such as our openness to a homosexual experience or a desire to have a little pain with our pleasure. We keep that stuff securely under wraps, perhaps never to be unveiled in our lifetimes. Or perhaps some of us unveil it in inappropriate ways with people who aren't our partners—and wind up getting ourselves in heaps of trouble.

When it comes to sex, what is normal? How would we even know what normal is when none of us is willing to talk about the thoughts or wishes we fear may be abnormal? As a society we devour any information we can find on the population's sexual habits and mores precisely because each of us is obsessed with answering that question: Am I normal?

We certainly don't pretend that our thoughts or attitudes are representative of normal. That was not our purpose in writing the book. We are simply trying to stimulate and simulate a dialogue on sex that we hope can be replicated in bedrooms across the country. If you disagree with some or all of our answers, that's okay. After all, we don't agree with each other on everything. But we do talk. Hopefully you can do the same with your partners and friends. Ask their opinions on these subjects; offer your own. As we found out while we were writing this, there's fun and fascination in discovering what your partners and friends think about sex. We even found new areas in our sexual relationship that we'd like to explore more together— areas that we had previously kept hidden from each other. That only makes our partnership stronger, more interesting, more stimulating. We hope it has the same impact in your bedrooms—and living rooms, and kitchens, and backseats, and patios (and all the other places where sexual exploration has been known to occur).

Happy journeys!

What Brothers Think, What Sistahs Know About Sex

The First Date:
Is It Ever Okay to Do It?

From a Sistah

My father's rules for his daughter's dating: Always meet him there, always secure your own transportation home, and never, ever show up for dinner without enough money to pay for your own entrée—because the last thing you want is to eat a good meal, have him foot the bill, and then invite himself up to your apartment for some payback.

Payback, of course, being some bonin'.

His rules, of course, were never quite passed along to most of the guys I dated—which, of course, meant that if they didn't know the rules, they damn for sure weren't going to obey them. It was no

> **Sex Tip:** While intercourse and even serious tongue wrestling might be off-limits on the first date, there is a surefire way of communicating your feelings in an intimate and memorable way: a big, warm hug. None of us gets enough good hugs during the course of our days. A hug can be quite sexual and arousing, but it is not as forward and presumptuous as kissing and petting.

wonder, then, that one way or another they'd find a reason to accompany me back to my apartment—you know, "to make sure you get home safely," they'd say, a look of pure concern invading their pupils—and then, just as quickly, find a reason to come upstairs. There was the "I want to walk you all the way to your door" one, the "I'm kinda parched—think I could come up and get a glass of water?" one, the "Can I come upstairs and make a phone call? The batteries in the celly ran out," one, and, my personal favorite, the "I have to pee" one.

Anything to get upstairs.

They seemed to know, instinctively, that if they made it past the first lock on the front door, they were going to get some. And if that could happen on the first date, hell yeah, they were going to take advantage.

Which, of course, we sistahs don't understand, because we know y'all definitely know the rule all of us women—whether we be black, white, American, Russian, straight, bisexual, virgin, or ho—have tattooed on the brain from birth: Do not sleep with a guy on the first date, especially if you want to see him again for something other than just sex.

This, for some reason, rarely stops you from trying, though. It is a rare man who won't push some button—whether in the pre-date telephone conversation, the talk over an after-dinner latte, the cab ride home, the doorstep kiss—that will get him into the door and will lead to his johnson getting wet.

And we're left trying to figure out a way to keep you from getting in—or figuring out how we're going to save face the next day after we done broke down and given you some on the first date (this, I would like to think, though, is extremely rare). I mean, it's not like we're not going to see each other again, right? If you like me enough to sleep with me, then you should be willing to wait—at least that's what we're reasoning when we tell you nicely but succinctly, "I really have to get to bed—alone—as I have to wake up early tomorrow. Got something to do—so, uh, good night."

And if you don't like me, then what the hell are you doing trying to sleep with me in the first place? Surely you can't be that desperate.

Basically, we don't quite get your sense of urgency—the thing in you that overrides all mode of sensibility and decency and leads you to believe that, if you try hard enough, you're going to get some from me, a total stranger. On the first night.

Excuse us—but chances are we probably don't know you from Adam. Why would we want to go there? I mean, you could be an ax murderer, a serial killer who ties women up, rapes them, then leaves them for dead. Or, you could be a serial screwer—screw her, then move on to the next victim, never quite settling down with any one woman, but quick to break hearts.

And if you know that we're thinking this way—and we know that you do, because there isn't a man on the planet who hasn't told his sister Fannie, his cousin Tammy, his friend Pammy, or his daughter Annie the same rule that we've been told practically every day of our dating lives—we're figuring there's no reason for you guys to be pushing us to have sex with you on the first date (or the second, third, fourth, or fifth for that matter).

Doesn't stop most of y'all, though. Why do guys push for sex on the first date—even though they know we've been told from birth not to give it up until later?

From a Brother

Because we've all been ruined by the little fast-behind girl in eleventh grade or sophomore year of college who shocked us by giving it up before we even figured out how to ask for it. We'll call her Keisha. (I've never so much as kissed any girls named Keisha, so don't get distracted by the name.) Keisha was so eager and she made this whole getting-into-a-girl's-pants thing seem so easy that we deluded ourselves into thinking they were all going to be like that. Lo and behold: They weren't.

But we keep trying, doggedly sustaining the flame of our prayer that we will one day meet another Keisha. We meet a lovely woman, she responds to us, we ask her out, she accepts, we do the dinner and movies thing, we have a good time, we're driving back to her place—and all along, prancing suggestively in the backs of our minds, there's Keisha. Keisha gave it up, right? Maybe this new woman is a founding member of the Keisha school of first-date bonin'. So we make enough entreaties, enough of a token effort, to give the new woman a chance to offer up the good stuff. Of course, we don't expect her to. In fact, we would be shocked if she did. We might even start wondering about her morals, or at least her past, if she did give it up so fast. Like in the movie *About Last Night,* in which Demi Moore has a one-night stand with Rob Lowe and then they try to forge a relationship afterward; we'd almost have to forget the first night happened if we're going to have the kind of respect for her that we'd need to have. But still we try, hoping that the ghost of Keisha inhabits her soul and she gives it up.

You wonder why we try, but you also know what happens to the brothers who lay back and never give it a shot, right? They get consigned to the "friend" category. In effect, they get punished for being courteous and respectful and so much fun to be around—the woman doesn't want to lose their friendship by sleeping with them. Ironically for the guys who find themselves in that situation, they were making themselves into such the good friend so that they could figure out a way to get into the pants. But, as Chris Rock says, they made a wrong turn somewhere and wound up in the "friendship zone."

There is one thing about Keisha that we can say with certainty: We'll never forget her. She stays with us forever, even after we've forgotten the name of that girl we dated for a few months freshman year or the one we made out with in the bathroom at that wild party senior year. Keisha has found a way into our hearts and heads permanently—whether she wants to be there or not. She's like our sexual muse, the inspiration we use when we're trying to get up the nerve to make that move or make our intentions known.

When I first started dating as an adult, the flirting and the sexually suggestive comments gave some form to the evening, providing me with a sort of script that I could follow to disguise my cluelessness. I usually knew I wouldn't reap immediate rewards, but I was planting the seed for future sowing. A few times, the future wasn't too far off—like the next date. One time, the future was the next date, on the way home, in the car.

By the way, though you describe our attempts to "push" for sex on the first date, I'm not so sure that that's what we're doing in many cases. If there's pushing involved, it's to see how far we can go. To see how much of our ever-present horniness can be relieved. If you reveal yourself to be open to some tongue wrestling, we're going to take that and see how much more we can get. Will she let me grope her breast outside her shirt? Yes? How about inside the shirt? Yes? Okay, how about inside the bra? Yes to that, too? Well, let's try to take the shirt off then and maybe suck on the breast. Yes to that, too? Well, damn! Maybe I can slip my fingers down inside her panties? Yes? Ohmigoodness! How about pulling the pants off? No! Okay, well, then I've found her first-date limit. I don't push it any further, I take what I've already gotten, then maybe I go home and finish off the job myself with the memory of that delectable-tasting breast bobbing in my head. As you're closing the door to send me on my way, you tell your girlfriends or tell yourself that I tried to "push" you into sex, whereas I walk away thinking that I got to suck your breast. The sex act itself was so far from happening that it hasn't even occurred to me as an actual destination.

Do women ever use guys just for sex, then discard them right afterward—even if it's been one date?

From a Sistah

All of us have had that one guy—that one with the conversation of a three-year-old, the sense of a billy goat, the sensitivity of Slobodan Milosevic, the face of Maxwell, and the body of Billy Blanks—that we've just gone on ahead and said, "Alright, screw it—I might as well bone him. He's too fine for me not to, and no one will ever know."

He's the funny bone of the skeleton in our closet—the one that we keep stored away to make us giggle. We know we took advantage of him, and he was too dumb to realize that the joke was on him, because, after all, he got some and moved on, too. We also know that there will likely be no consequences to deal with—because if it ever got back to anyone we know mutually, we could simply deny it and everyone who inquired would believe that we would never have done something like that because we're not inclined to be so stupid, so low, so . . . whorish.

The situation that puts us in this space is almost identical for most women; it starts with us seeing this hottie in his nice suit, on the way to wherever it is that he goes in the morning or at the club standing by the bar with his boys. He is fine. He looks like a matured Kobe Bryant, except his hair is combed and he got a little bit more meat on his bones.

He is, by all accounts, polite—a gentleman. He has communication skills enough to hold a decent introductory conversation, and, combined with a killer smile and a nice enough request, we are convinced that it is, indeed, okay to up the digits. We actually look forward to the call, and when it comes, we're picturing in our mind what he looks like as he's talking to us, if he's dressed or, um, um, um, undressed, sitting up, or lying down. We enthusiastically make plans to meet up with him somewhere, hang up the phone, and fantasize about how cool it's going to be to court, screw, then commit to this man.

Then the date comes.

He is a complete ass who makes no bones about showing his ass. He brags about his car, his suit, his titles, his house, his trips to Aspen—whatever material things he could possibly mention. Or worse, he has no car, you saw his one good suit, he lives with his mama, and he ain't been bold enough to pay $1.50 to venture beyond his Brooklyn neighborhood because he just loves Brooklyn so much he sees no reason to leave. I remember one of my girl-friends telling me about this one fool who had the nerve to ask her if her hair was real (it was) and then extol the virtues of natural hair, unshaven pits, and African attire over that "overpriced designer crap you women always want us men to buy you." Mind you, boyfriend was so worried about wrinkling his Armani that he could barely sit in his chair properly, and Mr. Natural had some kind of drip-drop mess in his hair, looking like a combination of Bill Bel-lamy, Ginuwine, and the S-Curl man.

She took him home and screwed his brains out.

It was good.

He left.

She never called him again.

Wasn't worth the time, energy, her hair, or all the African attire she would have had to import to her apartment to replace her clos-etful of fine clothing. Why bother, she figured. This definitely wasn't a love connection—not even Chuck Woolery could make this one sing. He wasn't her type; she wasn't his. It was obvious they had some serious philosophical differences—and that ol' boy was ready, willing, and able to be a complete control freak who would drive her batty, batty, batty.

That's all to say that not all men are worth the effort, and not all women are that desperate that they would try to turn every sin-gle date into a ring and marriage certificate. Some women do believe that it's okay to just go on ahead and get their groove on and move on; they just don't indulge in this as much as men do.

Nowhere near as much.

Why? Because most of us have been taught better than that—
or are just plain scared to do it. Those women will have their dinner
paid for, let him foot the cab tab, talk about him like a dog to her
girls, and refuse all phone calls from him—or simply pray that he
loses her number.

**If I gave it up on the first date, would I lose you? After all, I
could look at it just like you all claim to: We're adults!**

From a Brother

*No, you wouldn't necessarily lose me if I think that you're someone I'd
like to get to know a lot better and really enjoyed being around, but
you will make it harder for us to get past the monumental conception
I'm forming in my mind: The reason we get together is to have sex.*

Just as Pavlov proved with that dog, our minds are quickly
programmed to make connections. When we go out with someone
and a few hours later find ourselves deep inside her, that fact is
going to make quite an impression on us. We're not likely to forget
it. The next time we go out with her, we're going to spend much of
the evening thinking about it and waiting for it. Even when we're
not with her we're going to be thinking about it and waiting for it.
It's going to take a major effort on her part and ours to view our
relationship as more than a bone-fest.

What many women who have stumbled into this situation
decide to do is slam their legs shut and tell us we're not getting any
more because they want us to start seeing them as more than sexual
objects. Then they force us into those awkward evenings during
which we're supposed to discover all the other things we have in
common and explore how much we really appreciate each other in

nonsexual ways. But instead, what we're thinking about is how much we'd really like to treat her thighs like a juicy drumstick. It doesn't work. The couple of times I have been in this situation, the thought that coursed through my mind again and again in a closed-end loop was this: How can I get the hell out of here?

What needs to happen is that we get an opportunity to find out what kind of person she is without the sex distracting us right off the bat. We need to connect her to other things in our minds besides screwing, like how much we adore the way her eyes twinkle when she laughs or the cleverness of her sense of humor or the tilted but affecting way she looks at the world. Once impressions like these have a chance to form, then the sex will be buttressed by enough substance to keep us coming back even if we're not always going to end—or begin—the evening together in bed.

I know I have said in the past that men are capable of compart-mentalizing sex and the way we feel about a woman, putting them into two separate boxes. But if the sex compartment is nurtured and fed at the start while the other box is neglected, sex is going to loom as a monumental force in that relationship. If you then try to take it away to focus on the other things, you're going to find that there are not a whole lot of other things to focus on.

A lot of males are subconsciously aware of this when they go out on dates. Females might have a hard time believing this, but there are occasions when we find ourselves *really* vibing with a new woman, when we realize we're so attracted to her that we refrain from initiating real sexual contact on the first few dates. It's almost as if this growing relationship is too precious and delicate to risk messing it up right away with the sex thing. We want to let the pressure build up a little bit, to create sexual tension so thick you could eat it with a fork, to make the sexual act a culminating, crowning event for our developing union. I admit that this thinking doesn't come to us often. In fact, it may come only a few times in a lifetime. These are the women who eventually become our wives or long-time partners, the ones who bear our children and carve out sizable acreage in our hearts.

This is not meant to imply that it's impossible for a couple to have sex on the first date and build a substantive, long-lasting relationship. There are rare instances when two people vibe on so many different levels that they can effectively cram two months of dating, of relating, of connecting, into four or five hours of intense courtship that climaxes with some climaxes. When I was a senior in high school I met a beautiful girl at the University of Pennsylvania with whom I had one of the most intense connections I've ever had with someone. We didn't sleep together, but we felt like we knew everything there was to know about each other after less than a day. I wound up attending a different school and never saw her again after that weekend, but I will never forget her. And she taught me a lesson I never forgot: When it comes to matters of the heart, time is relative. Like a flower's bloom captured with time-lapse photography, it is possible for two months to be compressed into two days or even two hours.

We also know that sex is that much more fantastic when there's a base of feeling and intimacy, closeness and affection, undergirding the act. There's nothing quite so thrilling as the first time with a lovely woman with whom we are falling in love. We can almost hear the fireworks blasting and birds singing and waves crashing, like one of those over-the-top love scenes in a romance novel. It's damn good stuff, something most of us would be willing to make significant sacrifices to experience.

Second, we find that we want to talk and cuddle and hug when the act is over, instead of wondering why we suddenly find our heart cold and empty when faced with the prospect of having to roll over and face you again. It's scary how quickly that warm and lovely face, that entrancing and enthralling body, is transformed into the face and body of an unappealing stranger lying in our bed. Our mind can play dangerous tricks when it's working in conjunction with our penises. We can make ourselves believe anything if we are angling for the honey pot—like how much affection we have for this woman we just met, how much we have in common, how lovely she looks when she laughs. But only with the passage of time—at least a few weeks—do we find out if our feelings are real or just sweet nothings whispered in our ear by Jimmy (or in most cases, shouted in our ears, since Jimmy probably can't reach far enough to be whispering).

The First Time: Getting to the Home Run

From a Sistah

Sometimes we think it would be easier to steal the president's car and rob Fort Knox than to be so bold as to let a guy know that we'd like to have sex with him.

I mean, sure, we throw out the signs—invite him over to the house for dinner, invite ourselves over to his house for a game of Scrabble, wear something really, really provocative to a place where we're both going to be alone—but we'd never come right out and actually say, "Let's have sex."

> **Sex Tip:** Overwhelm your partner with compliments. If there's one thing that alleviates nervousness and inspires us to scale even greater heights of passion, it's knowing that our partner already thinks highly of the way we look, the way we kiss, the way we lick, the way we perform oral sex, the way we touch, the way we move, the way we are. It works every time.

Because you know what would happen if we told some man that we wanted to bone him: Just get us a pair of those screw-me stilettos, a leather micromini, and a nice cozy spot over there on the corner of Thirty-third and Eleventh, because we get the impression that you all would think we're nothing more than hos. Just sign us up for part two of HBO's *Pimps Up, Hoes Down.*

See, we're under the impression—shoot, have been taught all our lives—that you all need to make the first move, that that makes you feel like a man. And any threat to that need for you to feel like a man will not bode well for the person who issued the threat—not even some chick who served up her booty to you on a platter.

I'm not saying that you wouldn't partake of the platter, of course. Surely, if we're offering, you're not going to hesitate to eat and be merry. But tomorrow, if we just wanted to have lunch with you and continue to get to know you better and, perhaps, fall in love with you and have you fall in love with us, would we be able to?

I don't think so.

What would happen is we would put ourselves into the bone-buddy category. At least that's the way it seems to always go down.

Happened to me once. (God, I can't believe I'm about to write this, because I don't need to give my husband any more fodder with which to torture me. He's good at that. I'll have to keep it non-specific and spare so as not to have to hear it for the rest of my life.) Anyway, there was this really handsome guy that I'd seen around, and, for once, I was bold enough to ask one of my friends, who happened to know cutie pie, who he was. My friend's eyes lit up; it was her chance to make a love connection. Before I could grab her fast ass, she was out the door, snatching him up by the arm and leading him into the room where I was chillin' out. The introduction went over nicely; he seemed just as interested in me as I was in him. We found out we had a few things in common, including the neighborhood in which we lived. Before he could get the name of his street out of his mouth, I was calling him "neighbor" and inviting him over to my apartment for dinner. You know, the neighborly thing to do.

He readily accepted.

Slow down; I didn't ask him to sleep with me that first night. But I did within the first month that we were getting to know each other. I'd invited him over to my place again and cooked for him again and we were sitting in the living room just having great conversation and looking into each others' eyes and lightly touching each other—pretending that it was happening by accident. And it just slipped out of my mouth. "I want you to make love to me."

Needless to say, boyfriend didn't hesistate to get busy.

I told him what I wanted because it was exactly that: what I wanted. It didn't appear that he was going to make the first move—and I wasn't quite sure why. I didn't know if he wasn't sexually attracted, although all signs indicated that he was. I didn't know if he was just shy, although all signs indicated that he wasn't. I didn't know if he wasn't interested in me that way, although all signs indicated that there was a physical connection. Either that, or he couldn't get enough of my home cooking. But I was figuring that, after a month, he was coming around for more than just a plate of my famous chicken parmigiana. He just wasn't pressing it.

I wanted him to. And I didn't want to wait any longer. I liked him. I wasn't sure if I wanted to spend the rest of my life with him, but he was good company and would certainly make a good boyfriend, and it was simply easier for me to tell him I wanted to have sex with him than sit around waiting for him to make the move.

So I did it. And we *did* it.

And about five months later, he was gone. Didn't have any reason to leave, just told me he needed his space.

And I just knew that I was to blame, that I'd moved too fast—I'd messed up by rushing it.

Perhaps I'm wrong; I never bothered asking him. Just licked my wounds and moved on. But I never made the first move again—not like that. Now maybe this guy was an exception, or maybe I was reading him wrong. Perhaps something happened that had nothing to do with my being the aggressor. I have no intention of asking him, though. So maybe you can help me out: **How would you feel if I was the one to initiate our first time together?**

From a Brother

You do realize this is every man's fantasy, right? That some beautiful woman will one day walk up to him and drag him into her bed because she was so taken with his looks and sensuality that she just couldn't help herself. It's the kind of stuff that our best friend, the one who used to imagine himself as the playa president, always used to claim happened to him, but we never believed him because it never happened to us. So if you initiated our first time together, you would forever be our heroine; you'd make us feel like the coolest, smoothest, sexiest brother on the planet. We would like that very much.

We feel like we go through most of our days looking for the sign. In our earliest years, the sign is an indication from that cute girl with the adorable plaits that she doesn't really hate us as much as all the other girls pretend to hate the entirety of our gender. So we study her hard, watching for a twinkle in her eye and the telling smile before she throws us the big grimace and sticks out her tongue for the benefit of her girls, who are busy ensuring that their ranks stay closed and none of them ever does or says anything nice to a . . . ugh! . . . boy. We boys have our own appearances to keep up—we're not supposed to like the females very much either—but it's kinda understood that we're going to be selling out all over the place on the down-low.

In high school and college, the sign is that unmistakable body language we get from you—the way you seem to often be in close proximity to us when we're not expecting it, the quick little smile you throw us when we happen to look in your direction, the loud whole-body laughs we get from you when we say something remotely humorous. If you happen to drive by a high school, stop for a minute and watch how much physical contact teenage boys and girls manage to initiate, seemingly unconsciously but actually quite calculatedly. Girls will smack boys on the arm or shoulder, boys will get girls in headlocks or some other intimately violent position. Often they will appear to be fighting or wrestling, but really what they're doing is touching. Sexual touching is too frightening and taboo, so they get their kicks by disguising it with roughhouse play. That's an obvious form of the sign.

When we're all grown-up, we're still on the hunt for the sign. They get more obvious now—none of us has the time or energy to be messing around with headlocks. We're at the club or the bar or the restaurant or the workplace or the grocery store or the car wash, and we're looking for prolonged eye contact, a smile, and receptiveness to conversation, in that order. Those three things tell us plenty, but we usually need all three to get up the nerve to make our move—the first two without the third usually isn't enough 'cause this thing has no future if you're not going to let me talk to you. The receptiveness to conversation usually lets us know that you're available—as opposed to a married or attached woman with a wandering eye but who isn't interested in cheating.

If you are receptive to conversation, we smoothly entrance you with our wit and polish, and if we actually decide to go out on a date, the next sign is the real big one: When are you ready to do it? We become experienced over the years at watching for that one—hmmm, she's inviting me over for dinner at her place; she must be ready to bone. Hmmm, she keeps saying she wants to watch a movie on my extra-large forty-five-inch TV screen; she must be ready to give me some. Hmmm, she's asking me to give her a massage and she's spreading her body over the bed to receive it; oh yeah, she wants me right now. These are the kind of calculations we're making, the signals we're waiting for, the reactions we're gauging. That's the way it usually works; that's as far as the woman will usually go to help us out. However, if we're in our car on the way to your apartment and you lean over to say, "I want you to take me upstairs and make love to me," effectively cutting through the bull and the guessing and the wondering, we are probably going to explode from shock and excitement. It's the kind of moment we dream about but rarely does it happen.

When I was a freshman in college, there was a pair of lovely seniors who lived in the suite above the one I shared with three other freshmen. We were fairly typical, clueless freshmen, studying hard, playing hard, and always in search of female companionship. The relationship between the average freshman male and the average senior female barely includes enough acknowledgment or contact to call it a relationship. If they notice that we're alive we're usually happy and grateful, particularly if they're attractive.

Imagine the emotions that churned through me one day toward the end of the first semester when one of the lovely seniors told me that she thought I was sexy and that she was attracted to me. This was so far out there that I wouldn't even have dared to fantasize about it. She was beautiful and sexy and smart as hell—in addition to being four years older and wiser and more experienced than I. Has there ever been a greater gift handed to a college freshman? It only took a few minutes for our lips to meet. We soon became a hot item; I practically moved into her room. I'd sometimes entertain myself by stomping my foot on the floor to communicate with my roommates downstairs and remind them that I was above them, I was with my senior woman, and I was quite superior to them as the loverman.

Never did it cross my mind that my senior woman was fast in the ass or trampy for making the first move—rather, I thought she was bold and assertive and went after what she wanted, which in retrospect was a pretty apt description of her. (Though I'm sure a few of those derogatory thoughts about my girlfriend did occur to some of my female classmates, who didn't appreciate a senior woman swooping down and stealing from the already tiny supply of black male freshmen.) I'll admit that most of us males are probably too egocentric and self-absorbed to think that the woman who makes the first move is motivated by anything other than our animal magnetism and sensuality. It'd be unlikely for us to figure that she made the first move because she's a freak mama who goes around seducing men all the time—unless we had seen her in action on other occasions. There's always the girl in high school or college who seems to be with a new guy every week and we suspect it's because she's not shy about opening her legs. A part of us is appalled and repelled by her; another part of us is wondering if we'll ever get a turn. No part of us wants to stay with her any longer than it takes to hit-and-run.

What makes a woman want to have a sexual relationship with a man?

From a Sistah

For some sistahs, it's just pure, unadulterated physical attraction; she saw him, she wanted him, she boned him. For others, it's simply time; they've been kicking it for three months, he's hanging in there, she's going to give him some so that he'll continue to stick around. There are still more who go by the biblical sense of begetting someone—waiting until marriage because, hey, that's what the Good Book tells them they must do.

But I'll venture to say that there's a group of us who combine a little bit of the first two with a variation on the third. We recognize that he is physically attractive. This, of course, may come much later if he's not the best-looking man in the world; his cockeye and bubble head may grow on us—but this takes more, *waaaaaaay* more, than our having gotten used to looking in his good eye. He may have to have a lot more going for him, like a really nice body, or a really sweet disposition, or a really nice pocketful of money that he is extremely generous with—or, like, all of them if we're not too desperate. We recognize that the time we've spent together has moved us to another level—that we've surpassed the courting-and-getting-to-know-you stage and moved into the comfort zone, in which we're comfortable taking, like, a dump at his apartment. And though we have not waited until marriage like the Good Book tells us, we have fallen in love with this man and can picture ourselves married to him—and we will show him this by making love to and with him. (Yes, I recognize that this isn't what the Lord had in mind, but for some, it's close enough.)

It is these things that will make us want to sleep with you.

With Nick, it was obvious when it was time. I fell hopelessly, helplessly in love with him—with his intelligence, his sensitivity, his emotions, his gentlemanliness, his respect, his admiration, his wit, his ability to fall in love even when love, in the past, hadn't served him well. And the brother was—and still is—fine.

I knew that it was time when I started waiting, with bated breath, for his phone calls. I knew that it was time when I started thinking about him constantly—in the morning, late into the night, while I was out on interviews for the *Daily News,* while I was out with my girls, while I was at the vet with my two bad-ass cats. I knew it when I'd invite him over for brunch and we'd read the Sunday *Times* together and I couldn't concentrate, not even on the really interesting "Lives" articles and the recipe pages in the magazine. I knew that it was time when I couldn't stand not being with him—that his kisses and caresses just weren't enough.

That was when I decided I wanted him to make love to me and me to him.

And that is the way it usually works with the lot of us sistahs.

There is no specific time limit for this; it could take her five months, five weeks, or five days to feel like this about you. No woman is exactly the same, and neither are the men with whom they're contemplating sleeping.

It's, all at once, that complicated and that simple.

How can I make sure you come back again—that I don't feel like you hit it and ran?

From a Brother

Unless you're known as the campus ho or the office slut, we're not going to be interested in running away merely because we had sex with you and you initiated it. As I said before, we're going to figure you initiated sex with us because of us, not because this is something you make a habit of doing. We will come back again and again if we have decided that you're someone with whom we need to spend more time. If that's the case, there's no chance of your being a hit-and-run.

Though it may not always be so obvious, you're the one who initiates most of our sexual encounters anyway. It ain't happenin' unless you want it to happen and you let us know that it could happen. You know what I'm talking about here—you usually retain control over the event. If you want to bone, you're going to send us the subtle and not-so-subtle clues telling us to go ahead and make something happen. If you want to stop, you're going to tell us to stop. About the only thing we control is how long it's going to last—and usually we don't really control that, either: Jimmy does. Women always make it seem like men have so much power and control over the sexual event; we're never really sure what you're talking about—aside from forcing you, which is against the law, we have to wait on you before anything is going to happen.

So when you ask how we feel about a woman as the initiator, we think that this woman is just a more plainspoken version of what we usually encounter. Like my college senior girlfriend, she may realize that nothing will ever happen if she doesn't make the first move—or she may be tired of waiting for the fellow to pick up on her many signals. I'm convinced that men don't even understand a large percentage of the signals women send out. We think she's ignoring us; she thinks she's coyly seducing us with her shyness. We think she disses us every time we're in her presence; she thinks she's showing us how much she likes us with her teasing wit. Maybe these signals would work if she were trying to pick up another woman—that'd be an interesting question to explore with lesbians—but for the male species she might as well be sending out Morse code beeps 'cause we often don't get it.

As for the office slut or campus ho, our feelings about her tend to be quite complicated. We have a certain fascination about someone so overtly sexual, so seemingly interested in humping for humping's sake. We want to see what it's like, to see if maybe she done learned something from experience that the other girls—the nicer girls we take to the movies and hope for a handful of titty at some point during the night—don't know about yet. But she grosses us out at the same time. It may sound like that Madonna–whore dichotomy that feminists claim we force all women into, but I don't think it's that simple. We *can* make room in our thought processes for the possibility that nice girls will enjoy and crave sex. When we run into these girls, we don't force them into the whore box—

rather, we worship them. But it's the girls who publicly flaunt their sexuality and seem to want to define themselves as sexual objects that I'm talking about. We wonder why they feel the need for the show; we're turned-on by them, but we suspect that they're not all they may seem. Just as the bully may use size and intimidation to disguise the fact that he can't fight, we wonder if the temptress is parading her assets to hide something else. Because in our experience this kind of behavior from our women isn't normal—meaning this woman isn't normal. We may want sexy, we may want sensual, we may want attractive, we may want talented, but one thing we sure as hell want is normal. Normal isn't average or plain; normal is stable, reasonable, level-headed. Normal will listen when we tell her that her dress is see-through and therefore not appropriate for the family reunion. In other words, normal won't embarrass us.

Performance Anxiety: Ridding the Jitters

From A Sistah

From my diary, sometime in November 1994:

Entry 1: I am scared to death. It is only two days away—this wondrous experience. I've been replaying it over and over again in my mind. It's just sex, but in my heart, I want it to be so much more. And although Nick professes that it is much more than a simple "screw," I can't help but feel this way. What happens after it's over? I have to lay there and wonder if I slept with him too soon, if I moved enough or better than the last chick he had, if he wants to come back

for more, if he's going to call me tomorrow and come up with a reason why he can't see me anymore, or, worse yet, if he's never going to call me

> **Sex Tip:** Do it on the terrace, in the backseat, in the backyard, at the park, in the building foyer, on the elevator—anywhere that's unusual, out of the ordinary, so different from where you've ever done it before that your performance will be the last thing on your mind. Sure, you might get caught with your pants down, but you'll be wearing the biggest smile your face has ever seen.

again, and then refuse my phone calls. My God, I've let my heart over-take my common sense—my heart and my libido. Am I doing the right thing? Forget cold feet; I have blocks of ice at the ends of my legs. . . .

Entry 2: We did it, and I was nervous as shit. I hope it didn't show in my performance! It was, indeed, incredible—perfect motion, perfect harmony, together as one. He was a sweet lover, and he was hungry for me—almost as hungry as I was for him. But I couldn't help but be hungry, scared—shit, downright paranoid. I felt like I was plotting some massive mission to seek and destroy someone—but it was so right. He brought me a rose and I brought him a poem, a negligee scented with his favorite perfume, chocolate-covered cherries, and a picture of me as a little girl, cheesin'. He liked it a lot. I hope he got that each item represented a sense, and that I wanted him to enjoy them with me. I did feel sad at the end of the night, though, as he didn't want to sleep over. I immediately called into question my skills. I mean, why not stay over and hug me and kiss me and hold me through the night? Did I not get the job done? He says he has to get up early, and if he stays, he'll miss every appointment he has scheduled for the next week because he'll be too busy eating me up! Sounds good, but still makes we wonder if he's just trying to get away. The only way I'll be able to tell is by the strength of his hug tomorrow. I can't wait to feel his strong arms around me again. I'm stuck—nose open, ass out. What have I gotten myself into?

Entry 3: We did it again, and it was glorious. I wasn't anywhere near as nervous as the first time—and I didn't think it could get any better than that, but if this is any indication, we have no problem being sexually compatible. Ol' boy got skills! I've never felt so relaxed, so at peace with our relationship. We made love and lay in each other's arms, pigged out—enjoyed each other. The bath was the icing on the cake. He brought candles and we held each other in the water—talked about nothing in particular. He bathed me; I bathed him. I felt like a queen. I can truly say that after tonight, there is certainly no doubt in my mind that this is a special man I'm dealing with here, and I truly don't want what we have to end. He is my prince. . . .

Hell yeah, we women have performance anxiety—but it's, I think, different from what men face. You guys have equipment that could readily let your partner know you've got a problem; if Jimmy doesn't wake up—y'all got issues that will have to be addressed, and I guarantee you that as nice as she is when it happens, you will be addressing those issues on your own tomorrow. But for us, it's not as readily apparent—we can play it off, kinda. Nothing, after all, is going to refuse to work for us. If worse comes to worse, all we have to do is spread 'em and move the hips a little bit. But emotions don't, won't—can't—lie. We are tossing around in our mind all kinds of crazy thoughts—whether we're performing well enough, whether you noticed my padded bra was filling out that tight sweater the first time we met, whether my butt is big enough or my hips spread a little too far, how we stack up to the last woman you were with, whether you're enjoying yourself, and, the mother of all anxiety wonders, are you going to call tomorrow?

With all that on our mind, it's pretty hard to do what we're supposed to do—and that could leave you thinking we're boring lovers. In some cases, there might be some overcompensation—girlfriend may work it out even harder to make *sure* he's coming back. But the anxiety will still be there in the morning—with her worrying whether he's going to, well, come correct.

As we get more sexually experienced, we realize that you guys aren't the sex masters that you all proclaim yourselves to be. Sure, when we're younger and way more naïve, we actually believe all the hype you guys get by dint of just being guys; everyone assumes that you've been knocking boots since you were twelve, and that, at age thirty, you all know what you're doing because you've been doing it so long. Then we grow up and realize that just because he's been having sex since a young age doesn't mean that he knows how to screw better than the guy who righteously slept with only the four girlfriends he actually loved. In fact, ol' boy with the inexperience may be able to teach his hooker counterpart a thing or five more than he already knows.

All that's to say that as we get older, we do grow to accept that there may be some measure of fright with men—some kind of performance anxiety that accompanies your rolls in the hay. We recognize that no man is perfect. It's hard for us to tell, though, when he's nervous and is suffering a bout of performance anxiety, as opposed to when he just can't get the job done.

How do we tell if a guy is really just scared that he's not going to do the job right—as opposed to a guy with absolutely no skills?

From a Brother

The difference is quite clear: The Nervous Nellie might have been erectionally challenged that first time or two, but he's going to find a way to make up for it by using everything else at his disposal, like his touch, his tongue, and his imagination. The clueless brother with no skills is not going to be so proactive. He will become so obsessively focused on his failure, on the limpness between his legs, that he won't even consider doing other things to please the woman.

We've all been there. We meet a fine new honey. We kick it to her and we're thrilled to discover she's actually very responsive. She gives us all the right signals that she's down for whatever. We go out on a few dates and the sexual tension starts mounting like a tidal wave. We dream about her at night and all day. We try to imagine how her skin will taste, how those curves will look under our caressing touch.

A few weeks pass and, finally, the day arrives: It's bonin' time. As the date progresses, a whole lot of crazy questions start flying through our head. Our palms start to sweat. We sit back in wonder—and then it hits us: We're scared.

What if she thinks we're not big enough? What if she thinks we got no skills? What if some brother turned her out and she's expecting a cross between Moby-Dick and Superfly? What if our breath stinks? What if we forgot to change our sheets? What if we cum too fast? And the whopper, what if Jimmy fails to rise to the occasion—in other words, we can't get it up?

Because we all know that Jimmy has a mind of his own. He does not take orders well—in fact, he occasionally does the opposite of what we want him to do. And Jimmy is at his most temperamental, his most dangerous, when we are nervously about to go there with a new honey whom we desperately want to impress. Jimmy doesn't like it when we're nervous—he hates feeling that pressure. We know if he feels it, he just might rebel.

I can say from personal experience that there are not many feelings as sinking and scary as the one that infuses our being when it becomes apparent that the equipment will not cooperate. The first time it happened to me, I couldn't even look my partner in the face. The panic was so profound, so deep, that what I wanted to do most of all was flee. And, of course, the harder you try, the worse—the limper—it gets.

Eventually, what many of us learn to do in that situation is to let all that performance anxiety, that nervousness, work in our favor. We try to transform all that nervous energy into creativity. We know if we introduce other sensual pleasures into the mix, we will take all the focus off Jimmy—he won't feel like he's onstage anymore. If we do it right, she'll think we're God's gift even before she ever gets introduced to Jimmy.

God gave us the sense of touch because it is extremely important and powerful. When we start removing our clothes, we try to slow it down and explore with our fingertips. Every inch of skin that is revealed to us should become well acquainted with our fingertips before we move on. This might even encourage her to do the same. There is nothing more exciting than stroking and caressing smooth tender skin while concentrating on how wonderful it feels. That means we aren't thinking about how long we have to wait to stick it in; we aren't worrying about Jimmy's state of mind. We are staying in the moment and sinking into that exquisite tingle that has spread over our body from the work of her fingertips and ours.

After a solid ten or fifteen minutes of touching and stroking, hopefully she'll already be a quivering mess. But we're not close to done yet. Now our mouth goes to work. All those tender spots that received the benefit of our touch now get a loving visit from our lips and tongue. A kiss, a lick, a nuzzle with the lips and nose, even a deep, satisfying sniff of her intoxicating fragrance, everywhere. This is also not to be rushed. We won't even worry if she's now tugging at Jimmy like she's trying to draw milk from a cow. We're not finished yet.

The licking and kissing isn't done if we haven't gone downtown. We've heard the pleas of SWV, the harsh declarations of Lil' Kim, but brothers in the know have been performing oral sex for years—regardless of whatever stereotypes you've heard. As for technique once we get there, I'm not gonna go into detail. That's for every brother to discover on his own. But I do feel I should say a word here about female hygiene. If things don't smell right to us down there, like the expiration date was sometime in the early '90s, we have a couple of choices. We can immediately pull our head away and ask if she washed her behind, but that probably will mean the end of the fledgling romance before we even get it started. (If it's *real* bad, however, this may be the move.) We can hold our breath, take the plunge and come up for air as often as we can. If it turns out that we really like the woman, we can start taking matters into our own hands: We can start out our sexual encounters with a shower, grab a washcloth, drop to our knees and give ourselves a clean slate to work with. We can tell her we're a Teddy Pendergrass devotee, inspired by "Turn Out the Lights," and we are following Teddy's advice to take a shower together—"I'll wash your body, you wash mine, yeaahh." Otherwise, we might have to invest in a scuba diving course to increase our lung capacity.

Once we have stayed below long enough, we are undoubtedly going to have a very pleased woman on our hands. This does a few things: She already believes we are the man, so much of our performance anxiety should be relieved; if we know she's satisfied, we won't be stressin' Jimmy as much anymore, and he can just relax and do the job he was designed to do. Also, we probably will get the downtown bonus special: She'll feel she should return the favor. That'll certainly put a smile on Jimmy's face, huh?

Sometimes, even after we have employed these techniques and Jimmy is poised and ready, once he slips inside he loses his mind and ends the party before it starts. If we are having a really bad day, Jimmy might lose himself as we are slipping on the condom—of course, we *always* use a condom (see Chapter 5)—but hopefully he'll at least wait to be introduced to the good stuff. We do everything in our power to hold him back, but we're as effective as a point guard (or anybody else) defending Shaq in the low post. When this happens, we immediately find out what kind of woman we have on our hands. There are several varieties:

The Nurturer: She smiles at us, tells us everything was wonderful and she hopes she gave us as much pleasure as we gave her. She strokes our face and our chest, sighs, and says she feels grateful to have been with a special man like us. We know her performance is worthy of an Academy Award, but when we look in her eyes all we see is sincerity. If we get this response, we should ask her to excuse us as we run out to the store to purchase an engagement ring.

The Cold Fish: She is absolutely still beneath us, clearly waiting for us to get up. We push ourselves off and roll over. She asks if we can pass her the earrings she placed on the nightstand. She puts the earrings back on, gets up from the bed, and heads for the bathroom. Before she reaches the door, she turns back around and says, "I need a ride home." What should we do? Grab our car keys and sprint to the car so we can get her back home before she changes her mind and decides she wants to stay.

Iron Mike: We feel her hands on our chest and we find ourselves hurtling through the air. "Is that it, muthafucka?!" she growls in our direction. "What the hell was that? You can't hang? I knew you were gonna be a two-minute bruva, soon as you started doin' all that lickin' when I was ready for the bonin'. What's the matter, you gay?" When she's done, we feel like we just went a round or two with Tyson. We can't remember our name, we don't know what state we're in, we can't even remember what we had for dinner. If we are crazy enough to let this one stick around, we better keep her teeth away from our ears.

Can you tell when a man is nervous? What goes through your mind if he can't get it up?

From a Sistah

He goes for a lip lock, and ends up sucking my cheek? He's nervous. He tries to carry me to the bed, and trips over air? He's nervous. He reaches for the condom, and knocks over my glass of Chardonnay, then fumbles with the thing so much that he drops it before he can actually get it on—yup, he's nervous. It's no wonder to us, then, if he has a little trouble, er, rising to the occasion and/or finding his mark.

The first few times, that is.

See, we're figuring that you all are just as shaky about what's about to happen as we are. We figure you all *think* that we're assessing the package, we're assessing the foreplay skills, we're assessing your smoothness, we're assessing your strokes, we're assessing your tenderness, we're assessing your aggressiveness, we're assessing your ability to keep it going, we're assessing everything. The fact of the matter is that the first few times—the first time especially—most of us are too worried about our performance to really notice whether you're worried about yours, much less not taking care of business exactly the way you should.

This, of course, is contingent on the relationship we have with each other. If we really like you, we've taken the time to build a relationship with you and we want to make it work, we're probably going to be way more forgiving, way more willing to work with you—to take the time to figure out whether you were simply nervous the first few times, or you just don't have what it takes to spark our fires and hose us down.

The same applies to whether you can get it up or not. Sure, it's shocking when it happens; no woman wants to be in the situation where brotherman couldn't get an erection; we already know it's embarrassing for you—but it's equally embarrassing for us. The moment is extremely awkward; we don't know if you have a problem or if we caused it. All kinds of things will run through our minds—"God, did I not do enough to get him excited? Did my body turn him off? Do I smell? What did I do wrong?" We will guilt ourselves into thinking that this was our fault, not his—particularly if we really like him and want this relationship to work.

And we would invite him back for another try—a few more, at least, until we figure out whether he was just nervous that time or he really needs to invest in some Viagra stock. Because after a while, the nervousness disappears; we know what to expect from each other, we know what's up under the fancy clothing, we know what the necessary body parts look like and are capable of doing—

possibly what turns the other on. And we're figuring that three or four times into it, boyfriend should have long ago gotten over whatever it was that was keeping him from doing his duty. If it appears that he hasn't, then we know there's a problem and that it's going to have to be dealt with. How it's dealt with depends on the woman; some are willing to work with it, while others are more inclined to figure that they need to move on because the sex thing isn't going to work itself out.

Of course, there are the women who aren't even going to give you a second chance. Venture to say that they are the ones who hopped into the sack with you real quicklike, because all they were looking for was a quick bone. You were nothing more than someone she was sexually attracted to, someone who could fulfill her sexual needs until she found the man who could fulfill every inch of her relationship needs. You may have been a dull boy but a cute boy, nonetheless—worthy, in her mind, of a quick trip to the boudoir.

So you best perform.

Because she will call you out—maybe not to your face, but certainly to her girls—if you can't get it up, much less handle your business. She's not particularly interested in your feelings or your excuses, and she damn for sure won't be looking to give you a second chance to jack up the fantasy she'd worked out in her mind when she saw your fine ass at the bar. She may not be too ugly about it, but you can pretty much expect that her answering machine is going to be picking up her calls for the next few months, and that she's just been too busy to dial your digits to arrange a late-night drink.

I'd like to think those women, however, are rare. I think that a large percentage of us are still sleeping with men only after we've decided in our minds that he's worthy of it and that we'd like to see where this relationship is going. That means that if he wasn't able to do what he was supposed to do, we're not going to automatically toss him from the bed, make him gather up his clothes in his arms and kick him out the house, naked, never to be heard from again. We're going to work with him.

But maybe you could help us understand how we can better do that. **If a brother has performance anxiety, what can we do to make him more comfortable?**

From a Brother

Aside from the Iron Mike response I described earlier, the second worse response you can have is to internalize our failure, to think that it has something to do with you. That shows the kind of low self-esteem that sets off major warning bells in our heads because we know it'll eventually come back to haunt us—she'll be a clinger and need the kind of constant reassurance that drives us crazy. We're nervous, we're anxious about everything going perfectly, then we discover the worst—we can't get an erection, or we have our orgasm as we're putting the condom on. We feel awful already—we certainly don't want to hear the woman say: "It must be my fault. Maybe you're not attracted to me."

Let me say this: You'd have to be pretty damn hideous for us to fail to get an erection because you're not attractive enough. Usually, the fact that we're about to get some is plenty incentive for us to rise up, whether she looks like Janet Jackson or the bottom of

Janet's shoe. Shoot, we could probably rise up just thinking about getting some from the bottom of Janet's shoe. The point is, rarely is a woman's looks the cause of our impotence. Over the years many of us have slipped our thingies into some places we wouldn't be so proud to publicize. Even on those occasions, getting an erection was not a problem.

What we want is to see sensitivity. For some women this comes naturally. They see someone else in trouble or in distress and compassion pours forth instantly. At birth they were fitted with an abundance of the empathy gene and it has never gone underused. These are the nurturers, the women we'd love to see as the mother of our children, the ones we want alongside us when trouble sweeps through the house, when the mortgage payment is late or short, when our paycheck comes with a pink slip, when our child gets suspended for fighting. Knowing that she will be understanding and supportive becomes one less thing we have to worry about; we get a big window into those traits when we stumble upon erectile dysfunction, otherwise known as Mr. Softee.

For some other females, compassion and sensitivity come to them about as naturally as generosity infusing the soul of Don King. Their most common reaction to their man is blame and censure. They wake up in the morning wondering how he's gonna mess up today. Hostility and anger come so easily to them that they wouldn't be able to prevent at least a little from seeping into their attitude when confronted with a man who couldn't get it up. Their first thought would be themselves, how he was unable to please them, how he failed them. These are the women we want to avoid at all costs, though some of us wind up with them anyway. Sometimes it is exactly this hostility that attracts us, that makes us look at these women as a challenge, an obstacle to be surmounted. And once we break through, once we see that perhaps there's a more tender side that only we're privy to, we become seduced by the specialness of our status as the only member of the club. No one knows her like we do. No one sees her smile except us. That might be fun and intoxicating for a second—and then the hostility inevitably starts getting directed at us along with everybody else.

It's just a matter of a short time until we get it right. If things don't go perfectly the first encounter or two, we will soon overcome our anxiety, as long as we don't start feeling pressure build each time and it doesn't happen more than twice. After two times, it will take over our mental state and we will become so focused on the erection and so fearful that it won't come that Jimmy won't stand a chance. That is the place where no man ever wants to find himself. So if it has already happened once, our partners must bend over backward to ease any nerves and anxiety the second time. That means taking things *reaaallll slooooooooooowwwww*, not rushing into the sexual act but spending quality time on the kissing and the touching and the hugging and the caressing—you know, all that stuff that y'all like.

Talking About It

From a Sistah

Hell yeah, we women talk about sex. Shoot—Monica Lewinsky told eleven people about her escapades with the playa president, including her former girlfriend Linda Tripp and even her mama. The dress, the Oval Office, the phone sex—everything.

Us sistahs' mouths are just as big—trust me.

Surely you know by now: All of us women talk dirty. We twirl sex around in our conversation constantly. Incessantly. Conspiratorially. Over coffee, over dessert—at the hairdresser, at the nail salon, in the mall.

Sex Tip: Use the telephone. This is particularly relevant for those of us who initially might be a little inhibited talking about sex in a serious way. Of course, phone sex is a time-honored method of erotic discourse, but the phone can also be useful for married or cohabitating partners who need to discuss something that went terribly wrong or terribly right the previous night, or who'd like to invite their partner into opening up more about sexual fantasies anytime of day or night.

When's the last time you saw the cover of an issue of *Cosmo* or *Elle* or *Essence* that didn't have a story about "Getting Good Loving," "Giving Good Loving," "Twenty Ways to Please and Be Pleased," or "Having Great (Viagra-less) Sex"? I can't name too many of my girls who didn't scan *The Starr Report* specifically to look at the naughty parts, then compare notes with the sistahs to see if we've ever been as freaky as Monica and Bill.

It's sex talk. Scandalous in Washington, but not around our girlfriends. And these days, it's *waaaay* more candid than it was when Mom sat in the kitchen with her girlfriends and talked about this and that while the cookies baked. Thanks to Starr, even some of our moms are talking about (gasp!) *oral sex.*

We're nowhere as prudish. We talk about everything from how those pants are fitting around his butt to how the butt will look without the pants on—whether it's the size of the boat or the motion in the ocean that counts. Shoot—I can't tell you how many of my girls said they'd have done Bill—and how they're looking into the workings of that cigar thing.

We're just comfortable with one another like that. From the time we started comparing bra sizes in the locker room, we've known that our girls would protect our most intimate secrets, the girl secrets, like when we got our period or who we kissed first or whether we were going to give it up to that boy in our college physics class, the one with the pretty eyes, and whether it would hurt if we did.

When we got older, the conversation, of course, got a little deeper; it wasn't just about penis size and oral sex, but dating, romance, commitment, the ring, and everything in between. It's only natural, of course. As with anything concerning a highly technical piece of equipment, we women are completely baffled by how you men work. You guys are the eternal mystery, and no matter how the conversation starts—it could be about grocery shopping, toenail polish, fade cream, hell, anything—it will inevitably end up on you all.

I wrote a story once for the *Daily News* on this very subject, and celebrated advice columnist Dr. Joyce Brothers told me that we women talk about men incessantly because we're trying to discover through analysis "what a healthy relationship is."

"We don't have a pattern of what's a good relationship," she told me. "We watch soap operas, we can see how to decorate a room beautifully, and the information from talk shows you can use in a trailer park—but not necessarily in anything related to your life. So women talk to sort of explore why he doesn't call, how they can make him call, how they can get him to take them out again, how to get invited to his party. It's about finding out about his behavior."

But Lord knows we'd clam up faster than a murder suspect on *NYPD Blue* if a man were to enter the room looking for a little sex talk. Shoot—we'd rather cut out our tongues and paste them to our foreheads than have a candid coversation about sex with some man.

This, of course, is your fault.

We've been taught from birth that you just don't talk about sex with a guy, because if you do, he'll think that you're fast in the ass. It's that simple. We assume that the moment we even think about working our mouths to say something about it, your little wee-wee will get hard as a moon rock, and you'll spend the rest of the night trying to zoom yourself into our orbit. We, of course, will spend the rest of the evening fighting you off us because all we wanted to do was talk.

So we shut up.

And we talk to our girls.

But, you know, mom told us oral sex was nasty, too—and she turned out to be wrong on that one, big time. So perhaps you could straighten it out for us **If we talk to you about sex, will you think we're hot in the ass and looking to get some?**

From a Brother

You mean get into the real stuff with us? Talk about what you like and don't like? Ask us what we like and don't like? Reveal sexual fantasies to us and ask about ours? Discuss the individuality of eroticism, the all-consuming wallop of the orgasm? Sounds pretty good to me.

If there's one thing I've discovered as a grown-up male, it's that women spend much more time than we do talking about sex among themselves. I'm never really sure how many details you all offer up, but it's pretty clear that you allow the subject to be introduced and explored when you're with your girls. Men don't. We might make vague allusions to sexual matters, but we're certainly not going to share with other men what we do at home with our partners. It's information they don't need; the image of our lady in a sexual encounter doesn't belong dancing through their heads. So what we might do is mention something about Woman in general, about her peculiarities, her pleasures.

But rarely do we replace that generic Woman with a name. When one of us does slip up and offer too much information, start talking about specifics, about what happened last night or what our girl did to us last week, it's usually followed by uncomfortable silences, homeys looking at the ground or out the car window. Usually the subject is quickly changed—most likely by the guy who messed up in the first place. When slipups happen, the appropriate response is never clear. Should we ask follow-up questions, should we laugh, should we make little jokes out of the information? None of these seem quite right; with them all there's too much of a risk of offense. While guys might spend hours ridiculing each other playing the dozens, we never really aim to offend one another. When it does happen, it's usually followed up with an apology or an attempt to defuse the tension by claiming we were just kidding.

In fact, when we're young, the other guys can determine how serious a guy is about a girl by checking how quickly he gets upset or tries to change the subject when his girl is the topic of conversation. Another guy can get away with remarking that a particular girl has a nice butt or big tits if she isn't attached to any male in the group, but such a comment is totally intolerable if made about a particular dude's girlfriend or love interest. When a girl passes from distant physical specimen to love interest, we can all tell right away when her name tumbles from someone else's lips.

We're not really used to sharing details about the sexual life that resides in our minds. Eventually, after years of marriage, we might get used to talking about certain aspects of our fantasy life, but even then we don't share most of it—often because we're not sure how our woman is going to react. We kind of dole things out a little at a time, uneasily watching her expressions and listening to her responses to determine whether she thinks we're some kind of sexual freak. We don't get a list of the proper sexual fantasies and fetishes on our way up, so as grown-ups we can never completely shake the suspicion that there just may be something wrong, something perverse, something unusual about the things we like or dislike.

Imagine the joy of a relationship in which all that stuff can be freely discussed from the beginning. We go out on our first few dates and we're telling each other much more than our favorite sexual positions, which is the kind of lightweight stuff that we reach for when we call ourselves having an intimately sexual conversation.

"How comfortable are you with performing oral sex?" she might ask. "If you're not totally confident in your skills, I'll let you practice on me."

"Sometimes it takes me a little while to get revved up for a second round of sex, you know," he might tell her. "There are things we can do in the meantime while I rest and get ready to go again."

"During foreplay, it really pleases me if you spend a lot of time stimulating my breasts," she could tell him. "You can use your mouth and your hands."

"If you don't mind, could we try anal sex tonight?" he asks her. "If it hurts too much, just let me know and we can stop."

A couple who had this kind of free and easy rapport would have a wonderful time in the sack, I'd imagine. There would be little chance of either partner being left unsatisfied, and they wouldn't hesitate to sound the alarm if things were getting too boring or stale. But for how many of us does this kind of frankness come easily? We have been frightened for so long about talking sex with each other that by the time we become grown-ups these old closemouthed habits are deeply ingrained.

When I was writing about sex education programs in New York City for *New York Newsday*, sex educators often told me that it's the fear and inability of adolescents to talk about sex with one another that leads to so many incidents of teen pregnancy. That sounded strange to me at first, but I soon understood what they meant. The teenagers didn't have the comfort and the vocabulary to discuss foreplay, to talk about the many things they could do together to be sexually pleasured. They were afraid even to talk about their sexual fears because they didn't want their beaus to judge them harshly. So in the midst of all that discomfort, they went straight to the one sexual act they knew something about: intercourse. And, of course, they did it before they talked about birth control. The result? Parenthood.

Does talking about sex with your man turn you on? How about when you talk about it with your girls?

From a Sistah

Well, first we'd have to get past the notion that we can't talk to you guys about sex—which would be a feat in and of itself, but possible once we get to know you better.

And this, dear, is wholly dependent on you.

I mean, you all can hardly hold a simple conversation about what you did today, or why you wanted to beat the crap out of your boss. We say, "Oh, I heard you've got some stiff competition on the job," and you say, "Yeah," and I say, "You wanna talk about it?" and you say, "We just did."

End of conversation.

Now we're supposed to believe that you're really ready to engage in a meaningful gab session about sex? One in which you really listen to and care about what I have to say—and not just that it's going to lead to a roll in the sack?

Don't get me wrong; the sexy whispers in our ear—the ones where you tell me what you'd like to do to my breasts, or where you plan to put your tongue, or your fantasy about me showing up at your job in nothing but a raincoat, my big butt, and a smile—are indeed turn-ons. It represents a certain intimacy from our men that's extremely sexy to us. It's also a signal of something to come, a sign that, "yeah, buddy, it's on," that we're going to get turned-out and when it happens it will go down in history as one of those trysts that will probably never, ever be topped. Until, of course, one of us comes up with an even more creative usage for chocolate syrup, red pumps, and the recliner at the local Macy's furniture store.

But when we women talk about sex, it's not simply to get turned-on. It's to ponder—ponder how we can make it better, more exciting, more romantic, more meaningful. We want to talk about what it was like for you the first time and who was your favorite and whether it was the upperclasswoman who taught you how to move your hips like that or your first true love. We want to learn what you've learned, and share a few tips of our own.

And, above all else, we want you to listen to us so that you can figure out what pleases us, too. This is the true turn-on—when you hear what we have to say, and then you think about it and execute it lovely. The execution may not even have to come two minutes after I finish telling you. (In fact, it would be better if you stored it up for later so that we don't feel like you were half-listening, saying "yeah, yeah, yeah" in your head, and pretending you're really concerned about pleasing just so you can get to sticking it.)

That is what will get the juices flowing the quickest: A man who wants to talk and listen and be attentive to our needs and let us know what his are, without the pressure of having to hop to it right here, right this moment.

Now, talking to our girls isn't a turn-on—at all. We giggle and laugh and cry and wonder and advise and coach and preach and cheer one another on. But we do not get sexually aroused talking about sex with our girls.

What we do get out of it is confirmation: confirmation that we're not alone in our frustrations, confirmation that we're not the only ones not getting some or not getting it good, confirmation that there is another way to please and be pleased. We also learn—get ideas, you know? Like the creative things we've done with Jell-O? That may have come from one of the more explicit conversations we've had with our girlfriends.

You should thank them.

Meanwhile: **If I ask for what I want, will I be labeled bossy or too demanding—a drill sergeant?**

From a Brother

It all depends on how you ask. We're not comfortable with being ordered around, whether it's in the bedroom or any other part of the

*house. If the asking sounds too harsh and demanding, we'll resist—
out of the suspicion that in her request is a condemnation of our lovemaking skills. But if the asking is sweet and soft and entrancing, you
could probably persuade us to put on a dress and high heels before we
slide under the covers.*

A kind request is always going to yield better results than
orders and demands. Most of us are constantly on the lookout for
the diss. We look for it in the tones that our friends, bosses, partners, and children use when they talk to us or ask us to do things.
We respond to the tone more than the actual request. If it comes as
an order, I'm probably going to be reluctant to scratch your damn
back. But I'll suck your funky toes if you ask me nicely.

A former editor at *New York Newsday*, who edited the
columns of the irascible Pulitzer Prize–winning columnist Jimmy
Breslin, once told me that you could change virtually every sentence of Breslin's copy if you started out by telling him how much
you liked the piece and how brilliant he was. But if you didn't
sugarcoat the editing with any advance praise, Jimmy would fight
you on every word. Most of us, male and female, are like that.
Without any sugarcoating, we're gonna fight you on every word.

Don't get me wrong: There are plenty of women out there who
are bossy and too demanding. They can't seem to help it; they've
grown accustomed to making people jump at the sound of their
voice. They confuse bossiness with strength—if I'm not bossy and
demanding, people will think I'm weak and a pushover. But they
make things so much harder on themselves because their personality invites resistance rather than cooperation. The strong woman is
able to convince others to run through walls for her without ever

raising her voice. It's the weak ones who need to use the harsh tone and loud voice to hide their insecurities and weaknesses. (The possible exception to this theory is our mothers, who get what they want no matter what tone they use—though even with them I'd bet the meaner, harsher ones encounter more resistance from their children.)

I should say here that I've noticed a large market out there for the services of dominatrices, those scary-looking women who get paid to abuse men in sexual and not-so-sexual ways. Because my aim is to refrain from judgment about another's sexual preferences, I won't offer an opinion about the gentlemen who frequent dominatrices—different strokes, you know? But I will say this: A sistah would need to let a brother know up front about her dominatrix tendencies—otherwise there might be problems when she pulls out a whip and tries to lash his ass.

Words are a powerful aphrodisiac, particularly when they come from the lips of a loved one. I can't even effectively describe how horny I've gotten when my wife has leaned over when we were out together and whispered in my ear what she wanted us to do to each other when we got home. The anticipation was delicious. So was everything else.

No Glove, No Love:
Who's Responsible for Safe Sex?

Sex Tip: Have fun with the condom. Make a game of it. Go to the pharmacy together, march over to the condom rack, and buy three-packs of a wide variety of brands and textures. Then go back home and see if the two of you can distinguish between them. After the first go-round, maybe do some Coke/Pepsi style blindfolded taste testing to see if you or your partner can identify the brand that you just used. Beats Scrabble, doesn't it?

From a Sistah

I was so mad at that girl I didn't know what to do with myself.

See, she'd just met this guy—a really nice guy, but practically a stranger nonetheless. He'd taken her out a few times to dinner, the movies, a few jazz concerts. And she proclaimed herself so head over heels in love that she was, not even two months after they'd begun dating, flipping through bridal magazines, trying to decide what her girls would be wearing to the wedding.

I thought it a bit much even then; two months is not a serious determining factor for whether or not a person is good enough to buy a piece of furniture with, let alone marry. But then girlfriend, a thirty-something who'd already been caught out there with one child out of wedlock, picked up the phone, and gave me the ultimate shock.

"I need you to walk with me to the drugstore."

"Huh?" I asked.

"I need you to walk with me to the drugstore. I don't want to be alone."

"Um, okay." I hesitated. "But what you need at the drugstore that you can't be alone?"

Her silence instantly let me know what was up. Girlfriend was way past bridal magazines. She'd taken it a million steps further than that by lying down, spreading her legs, and having unprotected sex—putting herself at risk for deathly diseases and a lifelong commitment to two more people—her boyfriend and yet another child.

I tried to hold my tongue; she was, after all, a grown woman and a mother to boot, so I knew she didn't need my lecturing. She warned me that if I was going to give her grief over it that I shouldn't walk with her to the drugstore, either. But then homegirl flipped, talking about "if those two lines pop up, I'm getting an abortion."

"I can't have a baby with a man I hardly know," she said simply. "I've only known him two months."

I was, and still am, sickened.

I can't for the life of me understand how a grown person—a professional, a daughter, a mother, a friend, a person who should just plain know better—could lie down with someone she hardly knew, offer her body to him without protection, and then turn around and say, with certainty, clarity, that she would abort if she were pregnant because she didn't know him well enough to have his baby. Beyond that, I couldn't believe that this grown person—a professional, a daughter, a mother, a friend, a person who should just plain know better—could basically attempt suicide by lying down with someone whose medical history she just didn't know.

Dumb ass.

Apparently, the world is full of them. The barrage of statistics and threats and horror stories about people living with—and dying of—AIDS apparently has had absolutely no effect on a segment of our population. Countless boys, girls, teenagers, women, and men are having unprotected sex, not bothering so much as to even consider putting on a condom, let alone taking the pill or inserting a sponge or a diaphragm.

The result is the ridiculously high incidence of HIV infections and AIDS in our community. According to the Center for Disease Control and Prevention, African-Americans account for approximately 57 percent of all new HIV infections and nearly half of all AIDS cases—even though we make up just 13 percent of the U.S. population. AIDS remains the leading cause of death among black people ages twenty-five to forty-four.

It just doesn't have to be this way, but our ignorance makes it so. He says "it just doesn't feel as good," and he lies down, hoping he can dip it in the raw without hassles. She says she doesn't want to insult him by pulling out a box of condoms. "He'll think I'm hot in the ass, that I'm screwing all the time. Particularly if the box isn't new."

Hey, I was a young adult once. I knew the pressure of making the guy feel good and not pushing him to do something he didn't want to do. Admittedly, I took a few too many chances myself, none of which I will get into here because I don't want to bring up official black history and get my husband all riled up.

But I grew up, got smart, and armed myself. And the quality of men that I was dealing with didn't mind if I stopped whatever we were doing to whisper, "Baby, go look in the medicine cabinet and get a condom."

Basically, I haven't come across too many men (well, I haven't had all that many, but still) who put up a fight to have unprotected sex. But as I understand it from a few of my girlfriends, my world is pat and limited. Men, they argue—particularly black men—would rather pack their own or take their chances. They damn for sure don't want you pulling out the box.

I find this hard to believe, but that's just me. Here's one chapter that the sistahs and I are going to argue over for life. Maybe you can clear it up for us: **What do guys think when a woman pulls a box of condoms from her drawer?**

From a Brother

When she reveals her own condom supply, we are definitely faced with one undeniable fact: We are not the first explorers to plant a flag in this hallowed earth. This fact is particularly inescapable if the box is a twelve-pack with only one or two lonely condoms left. And the fact is dramatized with bold-face exclamation points if this nearly empty box looks so crisp and new that the missing condoms had to have been used in the past seventy-two hours. However, being con-

fronted with evidence of her previous, uh, activity, though startling and memorable, shouldn't be a deal killer.

First, unless she's so young that we can still smell Similac on her breath—and if she's that young we shouldn't even be close enough to smell her breath anyway—it'd be downright juvenile of us to expect that in the year 2000 a grown woman is waiting until marriage to give it up. That kind of chastity has gone the way of the 8-track tape and affirmative action programs. I'm not saying that there are no recorded cases of adult virgins in the United States in this new century—I'm just saying finding one would be about as probable as Lil' Kim winning an NAACP Image Award. So even if our first reaction to the sight of her condom box isn't exuberant joy, it's not likely going to deter us from the task at hand.

In fact, it is the sistah who would let us in unsheathed who should give us pause. She's the potential trouble because if we're getting this kind of unfettered access, no doubt others have gotten there before us. Maybe enough others that we should be worried about our health and even our life. I don't think enough brothers go through this thought process, so intent are they on striving for the best possible sensation, for the most intense friction they can find, that they thrust first and ask questions later. In the early stages of a budding relationship, should any of us really think we're so special and so incredibly meaningful to this woman that she's going to give it to us raw, never having done it this way with any brothers who came before us? I don't think so. I think women who are in the habit of denying love without a glove are not going to suddenly lose their heads at the sight of our wonderful body, no matter how fine and sexy we are. But the women who are going to let you in without a condom are likely the same lazy women who haven't always taken the proper care in the past and insist on gambling with their safety and the safety of all the brothers they invite into their beds. Sure, these risk takers might use a condom sometimes, but sometimes just isn't good enough, is it?

A woman with her own condoms has two traits that should be important to most brothers: She's well prepared and she cares about herself and her future. In my experience, women with these traits are the kind of women I like to keep around. They're the ones who are going to have the address to the restaurant if you forgot where it is, who will have the pack of breath mints as you're walking up to her parents' front door, who will have an extra twenty dollars for the cab if you can't find your wallet, who will know exactly what to say (and what not to say) if you didn't get the promotion you were counting on. And if she cares about herself and her future, she's not going to be overreliant on you to provide her with the things she wants out of life—she's going to be out there trying to get them her damn self. In other words, this sistah is marriage material.

I might add, however, that we don't want too much preparation and too much concern for herself. Taken to an extreme, that translates to self-centeredness. So if the sistah starts shouting out directions as if we're a mere stagehand hired to do hard labor in the drama that is her life, we're probably going to leave skid marks as we dash to the wings before the end of the first act.

This whole question should be a moot point anyway to us righteous brothers: We should never get to the point where the woman has to pull out her box, because we should have our own.

And unless the whole encounter is a shocking surprise (by that I'm talking about something on the scale of Janet picking us out of the crowd and inviting us back to her hotel room, not "Well, it was just the first date . . . "), we would never be caught in an intimate situation without one. Right, fellas?

How long does it take for you to feel comfortable enough with a guy that you won't require a condom?

From a Sistah

The sane, rational, intelligent answer should be: after the negative results from the HIV tests come back, you two have said, "I do," and you've decided to start a family.

But that isn't realistic. Most people, even though they are about to perform the most intimate act anyone could ever perform with another person, are too scared—and too stupid—to ask someone for their HIV status before they lie down with each other. Most are also too hot in the ass to want to wait until they're married to sleep with someone—and hardly anyone these days holds off on sex until it's time to have kids, save for, like, Hasidic Jews. A lot of those same people who can't wait for the results, the ring, or the kids will also find an excuse for why they can't wait until the condom is on—and that's scary.

These days, condomless sex doesn't seem to be as prevalent as it was when I was in college back in the late '80s. The AIDS epidemic was just making headlines, and most of us were still ignorant about how you got it and what the symptoms were for those who might have it. So my friends and I were walking around saying stupid stuff to one another, like "Oh, he got a big cut on his leg during the football game and it healed up nice and quick, so he must not have AIDS," or "He doesn't *look* sick," or "Men catch that stuff from other men, and I know my man is *all* man, so he *can't* have it." We'd pop our pills or insert our sponges—because you know if any of us turned up pregnant, our mothers and fathers would have made sure we were dead, *dead, DEAD*—and go on ahead and lie down with the boy because we figured we were taking express measures not to get pregnant and that was the best any smart college girl could do.

It didn't take me long before I figured out that the pill was having serious adverse effects on my body, and I didn't trust my skills with the sponge or the diaphragm, so my safe-sex choice quickly became the condom. I knew that without the condom, I ran the risk of pregnancy, so it was a rare privilege for any man to get the opportunity to have sex with me without one.

In fact, only one man had that opportunity—and, at the time, there was sound reasoning for it: I knew that if we did get pregnant, he would be a great father to our child.

That's been my standard for a long time now: no glove, no love, unless you are daddy material. I wasn't trying to hear the "it feels better without it" argument, or the "I'll pull out in time, I promise" argument or any others, for that matter. In fact, if I heard either of those or "don't worry—you won't get pregnant," I'd run screaming in the opposite direction because that usually meant that this Negro standing before me was trifling as all get-out, and irresponsible to boot. He easily displayed that he was all too willing to take chances with his life—and mine—and that he wasn't thinking past the next thirty minutes he'd be having sex. The last thing a trifling, irresponsible man can be is a good father to a child.

He'd have to get up out my face. Quick.

Later on, as I began to fully understand HIV and AIDS (particularly how easily it could be caught and spread), even those who were deemed good daddy material had to wrap it up. I, after all, had a life to live, a lifetime to look forward to. There were so many things I wanted to do, so many things I'd yet to experience, and I'd be damned if I was going to miss out on any of it by needlessly giving myself a disease that would cut life short. If I was going to die, it was going to be because God willed it, not because I was too stupid to protect that which is precious: life. That sensibility, coupled with my absolute need to have a baby *after* marriage and not a minute sooner, meant that I was going to have protected sex *every time*. Shoot, I didn't even sleep with my husband without a condom until we decided it was time to bring another life into this world—and I had already married him!

And that's the way it should be with all of us sistahs.

I don't think any of us should take our lives into our hands and sleep with any of you without a condom until we are absolutely sure you don't have any life-threatening diseases *and* that we are ready to be a mother to your child. It's the really dumb one who will use neither a condom nor other protection when she lies down with a man—and every one of you should be wary of her. She's the one who will take yo' ass straight to court for child support, won't let you see your kid, and will hound you for the rest of your life.

But there are some sistahs who fall in the middle, who will sleep with a man condomless if they're in a committed relationship and she's sure he's only sleeping with her. That requires trust—and you would have to earn it before she decided it was okay to lie down with you unprotected.

I still maintain, though, that not even that is worth it.

That doesn't stop some guys from using that tired-ass argument, it feels better without it. Frankly, I've never really understood what was meant by that; to me, it just doesn't feel that much different. Help me understand: **Does it really feel different without one?**

From a Brother

Yes, it most certainly does feel different. There's just no comparison. It's like wondering if the food tastes different at McDonald's and a famously lavish restaurant like New York's Union Square Cafe. Of course, the food is immensely better at the latter—it's supposed to be. Otherwise a thirty-dollar entrée wouldn't make sense. Similarly, flesh-on-flesh sex is going to feel immensely better than trying to feel through a layer of latex. Since my sexual coming-of-age came in the early '80s, after the discovery of the AIDS virus, I automatically associated intercourse with condoms. The first time I had sex without one, I couldn't believe how much more intense and pleasurable it felt—because it had felt pretty damn good with the condom. But whether it feels different isn't the key question.

The key question is whether we're in the proper position to reward ourselves with that ultimate pleasure. It's not something that's just handed to us indiscriminately. We have to work toward it. In other words, we have to have put the time and effort into the relationship so that the woman trusts us and knows we care for her enough to take the risk of tossing aside the condom. In this age, this kind of trust isn't something we should take for granted. Consider how we get to that trust:

1. We must demonstrate to her the kind of responsibility for our actions and for our commitments that shows her we're somebody who will stick around for a while and somebody she can count on when her road gets bumpy.

2. We must be monogamous. After all, that's the point: If she's letting us come inside unprotected, she's showing us that she knows we haven't been sliding into any other places. If we have been, particularly if we have been cheating without a condom, we're putting this woman in danger of contracting a whole lot of problems she didn't ask for. If we have been cheating, we're proving that we're not ready for the unprotected sex.

In other words, if we're not going to be faithful, then we're not deserving of the love without the glove.

There are many times in our lives when we have to forgo or postpone our pleasures for the greater good. For instance, when we were little boys and we had to study for a big test the next day, we knew that we had to ignore the desperate calls of our little homeys outside—the same little homeys who failed the test and are now standing at the intersection asking you for change when the light turns red. When we first got the job and were rewarded with the early Saturday morning shift, we knew we had to cut short our Friday night partying so we could get home and hit the pillow.

After we got married, we knew we had to squeeze shut our eyes and ignore the entrancing booty and come-hither smile of the temptress in accounting—unless we wanted to witness our spouse transform into Mrs. Lionel Richie.

We learn to postpone our pleasures until we're in a position to receive them. Safe sex is the same way. Unless we've put in the work, we better slide on the glove and shut up.

Date Rape:
When Does No Mean No?

Sex Tip: Antioch College received a great deal of attention—mostly negative—in the early '90s with its alarmingly didactic sexual harassment policy intended to prevent date rape by forcing students to get permission before proceeding with each step of a sexual encounter. Faced with a circumstance in which consensuality is unclear, you could use the Antioch College Sexual Offense Policy and make it work for you. The policy can be your road map to sensual delights,

From a Sistah

She was there for the same reason everyone else was—a little nightlife, a little partying, free booze and chips, the cute jocks. She figured it was safer to avoid the bar that night; she'd heard so many horror stories about girls going over to the local college hangout, getting drunk, leaving with some guy, then being invited on a "train ride" they didn't want to take and forever paying for it with years of pain, nightmares, and, worst of all, "she's a ho" rumors.

So she called around to find out where the dorm parties were and found one in a building not too far away from where she roomed. It would be safe, she figured; she'd take her girlfriend—that chile never passed up a free drink—with her, she knew a few of the guys who would be there, and the residential assistant would be just down the hall in case things got out of hand.

The party started out relatively calm for a college get-together. The music was pretty low, everyone had a drink in hand, but nobody was hooting and hollering like they usually did at these kinds of get-togethers. A few of the guys, boozed up, were trying to play a game of spades; but, as you can imagine, it wasn't quite working out since, in their drunken haze, nobody could quite get that the spades trumped all the other cards. It wasn't too long after that that her girlfriend started giving

allowing you to get thrilling little green lights from your partner at every erotic intersection. **Note: As you move to each new step, your questions must be posed seductively in your best Barry White voice.**

YOU: "Baby, can I fondle your breast, baby?"

YOU: "Mmm, that's nice, baby."

YOU: "Baby, may I take off your bra, baby?"

YOU: "Oooh, baby, I looove the way it feels to me, baby."

YOU: "Baby, may I kiss your nipple, baby?"

YOU: "Shaw nuff tastes gooood to me, baby."

You get the idea.

the eye to her ex—and her ex started giving the eye to the other guys. One by one, folks started filing out—stumbling out, really—each of them getting the hint that some sexual tension was in the

air, and some bonin', or at least heavy petting, was about to commence. The girlfriend realized, however, that she was too drunk to
make it back to the dorm by herself, so she asked her friend to
stay, to wait on the other side of the room (it was divided into two
separate spaces by two huge movable closets to optimize privacy)
until she was ready to go. She agreed; the bed over there looked
plenty inviting to her woozy eyes—about the only thing in the
room that wasn't spinning. She sat on it and looked out the window, trying to block out the sounds of lips smacking and hands
connecting with skin and unzipping zippers on the other side of
the room.

She barely noticed him when he walked in, this beautiful speci-
man of a man. He was a football player, one of their best, and the
muscles that bulged from his T-shirt easily alerted anyone looking
that he spent quite some time in the weight room—this much she
knew. He was good-looking, too. And it didn't hurt that he was talking to her real soft and nice—not those smooth-daddy lines, just real
normal-like—or at least let the liquor tell it.

Before she knew it, they were wrapped in each others' arms,
kissing and hugging and touching.

Before she knew it, he was tugging at her zipper.

Before she knew it, he'd ripped the delicate material that held
her lace, french-cut panties on her body.

Before she knew it, the word "no" that had slipped so delicately,
softly from her lips just a few moments before was now becoming
more frantic, more desperate, louder.

No one heard her.

He certainly didn't act like he did. And if he had heard her, he ignored her.

The man that she had willingly kissed, touched, and caressed—but didn't want to sleep with—raped her.

And the next day, when she got up enough nerve to say what happened to her, almost anyone and everyone who was listening (save her girlfriends, who all knew her better) said, "Sounds like consensual sex to me."

It is a classic example of a date rape. What she thought was going to be a round of petting turned into something she didn't want. And no matter how much she said no, no matter how much she pushed and shoved—no matter what she did to stop it—he wanted it, and he took it. Sure she kissed him. Sure she touched him. Yes, she was drunk. But she didn't want to "do it."

He, on the other hand, took her drunkenness and her willingness to kiss, caress, and touch as a sign that she wanted to have sex; and when the light turned green in his eyes, he proceeded to go. Emergency alarms be damned, he was behind the wheel and he was going to proceed.

Ironically, it seems that a majority of the male society would agree that he had the right-of-way here. She willingly kissed him. She willingly touched him. She willingly hugged him. How on earth could she not have been willing to go all the way? She was drunk; she probably doesn't remember how much she was turning him on, they say. Women who turn to law enforcement (most of them men with the same jacked-up attitude) are told to "just forget about it."

And the women who were violated are forced to deal with it alone—their attackers often moving in the same circles as they— forever, if they don't seek help, jacking up their relationships with other men. Either that, or they simply convince themselves that it was their fault and move on. (In her case, because she could get justice from neither the university nor the local police department, she had a few of her friends kick his ass. Hard.)

Sure, all of it could have been avoided if she had simply told her friend she wanted to go back to the dorm. Sure it could have all been avoided if she hadn't kissed him. But it also should have been avoided when she said no.

Problem is that too many men, it seems, don't understand the word "no." Can't count how many times I've heard some dumb-ass man stand up and say—without laughing, serious as cancer—that sometimes, "no" really means "yes."

"She's just saying that because it looks better—makes her feel like she's not a complete whore for agreeing to sleep with a guy so quickly," they say, unflappable.

This may not happen as often when we get a bit older and totally out of the college scene, but there is a long period there where we women have to deal with you guys' stupid justifications for why you've basically committed a felony and gotten away with it. You all may forget about it two days later, but we women are left to deal with it for the rest of our lives, always wondering if this thirty-year-old, forty-year-old, fifty-year-old man whom we've invited to the house for dinner and candlelight will instantly revert back to his teens and forget that "no" really does mean "no," and try to test us.

For us, it's an issue of safety, part of the reason why we don't talk to you on the street, why we go to public places for our dates, why we won't let you into our houses at the end of the first date— even if you swear you just want to use the bathroom. It's sistah defense, because we know your no-doesn't-really-mean-no argument could creep up at any time and render us completely, totally helpless.

There are even times after we get with a guy—after he's earned our trust—that he'll trip and continue to head toward the hickey, even when we've told him he shouldn't. You all claim that if the vibe isn't right, you'll leave it alone, but it seems that if we show the slightest hint of romance, "no" isn't really good enough unless followed by a billion others, most of them with bass in the voice and a whole lot of attitude. She may not have to beat you off of her, but— mentally exhausted from worrying whether you're going to stop or not—you two might as well have gone twelve championship boxing rounds.

It is, indeed, tiring to have to constantly think about it. But we recognize it's necessary.

Why is it that we sometimes have to say "no" a billion times and, in some cases, fight you before you recognize we don't want to have sex with you?

From a Brother

Fight? Speaking for myself, I'm out the door and back on my horny little way long before the sistah feels like she has to take a swing to keep me away. I would hope that the majority of brothers feel the same way I do. For us, there's too much pride and ego involved in the sex act (perhaps, at times, unfortunately so) to keep pushing a woman well after she's made it clear she doesn't want our sorry behind. But I suppose there's a destructive and dumb minority of brothers out there who blindly forge ahead, even after the woman is crying and perhaps screaming—they're either not picking up the signals that are as obvious as the empty space between their ears or they haven't thought ahead to consequences beyond the damning inevitability of their ejaculation.

In our adolescent and postadolescent years, however, even for those of us who'd never think of committing a rape, the confluence of girls and sex can sometimes get confusing as hell because of the usual presence of that liquid sorcerer: alcohol. It is the social enabler of choice for many young males and females, allowing us to shake off our inhibitions and do all the things we secretly covet yet fear. Often, that means having sex—particularly for the females.

In high school and especially in college, I'd watch the girls throw down glass after glass of alcohol and then disappear with one fellow or another—a few times, I was even the beneficiary of their newfound enthusiasm. We'd wander off somewhere and something might happen or it might not, but I always got the impression that the girl needed the alcohol as a motivator. On one occasion, a thoroughly intoxicated college classmate who seemed quite eager to be alone with me suddenly stopped the proceedings, as if a voice managed to fight through the haze to tell her she was going too far. So we stopped. There may be a few guys out there who wouldn't have stopped under those same circumstances; they might have figured that since she practically dragged them into the encounter she didn't really want it to end and was only protesting because she thought that was what was expected of her. But the woman has the right at any point during the tryst to change her mind—that's what the law and common decency tell me.

Yet I've also had a few debriefing conversations with women who have said that even though they told me to stop and a part of them clearly wanted me to stop, another part of them wanted me to ignore their STOP sign and keep going. It was almost as if they wanted me to take responsibility for what happened, even if they really wanted it to happen, so that they could retain their chastity and still have sex. This is some complicated stuff; many guys, upon hearing a confession like that, might take it as a signal for them to ignore the next woman's protestations, even though this woman may seriously want them to stop.

It may not be the most politically correct point to make, but guys have their own vulnerabilities when they go into that room with a woman they don't know that well and close the door. There's always a danger that she might not appreciate what transpired—or have some type of master plan at work—and come out of the room yelling rape. How many professional athletes have been caught in these predicaments, their names plastered across every sports page and television broadcast in the country, only to find out later that the woman made it all up in an attempt to get some cash? Or the female who gets caught cheating on her husband or boyfriend and concocts a rape story after the fact? There are enough of these stories in just the history of the American South to fill up a textbook, with the explosive element of race and racism often thrown into the cocktail to singe emotions.

I'm not trying to imply that the huge majority of rape claims aren't legitimate; I'm just saying that the question of consensuality can be a dicey one. Rather than trying to dissect the woman's state of mind and analyze the sincerity of her sudden rebuff, I have always thought it a good policy to retreat immediately upon hearing anything that sounded even remotely like a "no." That way, if you have somehow misread her intentions, she can let you know—or maybe she won't ever let you know. Either way, every male needs to realize there will be other opportunities, other women who will be much less conflicted about what they want to happen. Some of them won't even need alcohol to help them along.

Why does alcohol so often seem to be involved with your sexual encounters—especially in your early years?

From a Sistah

Crazy, isn't it? You'd think we'd know better—there have been enough after-school specials, Sunday night movies, and freshmen lectures to warn us that alcohol is the root of all evil on the college campus when it comes to hooking up with the opposite sex.

But it doesn't stop us.

I can't speak for everybody, but I can recall what was going on in my college experience. There's a party, it's supposedly full of cute guys—or at least the one she's attracted to—and she's just got to get over there to be in the same room as them or him, and make herself look as cool as possible to get his attention. That means she's going to talk about the party all day long to her girlfriends—on the telephone, over lunch, between classes. Then she and the girls are going to meet up a few hours before the big shindig and spend that whole time primpin' in the mirror, getting the hair, the outfit, the Maybelline just right.

And they'll walk to the party like sheep being led to the slaughter.

"Uh . . . hey, ladies," the cuties will say when they see the girls walk into the room. The boys will lead them right on over to the corner of the room where all the alcohol is, and encourage—in some cases, implore—them to have a drink.

The majority of the girlfriend crowd will readily drink up. They've been looking forward to the cocktails some guy will make up for them, with crafty names like Kappa Punch and Phi Ep Brew. It will have sat in a great big ol' tub for days—a bunch of fruit just drowning in vodka and rum and any other eighty-proof drink they could fit into the bucket. "Go ahead and have some," he'll say. "You can't even taste the alcohol."

And he'll be right. Before you know it, the girls are plastered off of fruit punch. And the few girls who didn't want to drink are being cajoled into taking a sip by their drunken friends. If they don't, they risk being teased for the rest of the night as "prudes" who don't know how to have fun.

And they will drink, too.

And sooner or later, all of them will be drunk off their asses, and the vultures—the guys looking for the end-of-the-night kill—will swoop down on the most vulnerable ones, the ones who can barely walk. And before you know it, they will commence to boning.

Peer pressure is a mug.

And I can't imagine that it's changed all that much since I was in college.

This is what it's all about, you know: peer pressure. We're pressured by our girlfriends to go to the party, we're pressured by our girlfriends and the guys to drink at the party, and we're pressured, again by both, to leave with the guy who's showing us a remote interest. And, in our drunken stupor, we'll go with him, completely vulnerable to this big, strapping guy who can overpower us, take us, and rape us at his whim.

At the root of it all is alcohol.

I don't think there's any coincidence that a lot of the cases involving date rape also involve drinking; you lose your faculties and find yourself doing stuff you would never do when sober, in situations you would never be in had you not been inebriated. Rest assured that a large percentage of women who are violated while they're drunk wouldn't have even been in those stupid boys' rooms that late at night without backup had they not seen the bottom of that tequila bottle.

But the one thing that always irked me most was the guys who pressured the girls to drink, convinced them to go back to the room, and then took advantage of them. I know that a lot of times, they, too, are under the influence of alcohol, but it's no secret that guys can hold their liquor more easily than women can, that they are stronger than women are, and that they are, more often than not, able to score—whether she is with it or not. What I cannot understand, though, is why there are so many young men out there willing to take the chance—that she will, the very next morning, find herself sitting in front of the authorities, talking about how he raped her. Surely, with all the publicity surrounding hundreds of college-age men being accused of raping acquaintances, you'd think guys would protect themselves and avoid those kinds of confrontations by waiting until she's no longer drunk to get some.

What possesses guys to be so stupid as to take a woman against her will without realizing that the consequences may be—or at least, should be—severe and quite unpleasant?

From a Brother

Perhaps it is because many times the consequences aren't severe or unpleasant enough. If guys didn't think they'd get away with it, I don't think most of them would do it. I've often heard it said that the only thing that prevents many people from committing crimes is the fear of getting caught. In other words, if put in a situation where they'd be assured of getting away with it, many people would steal the car, cheat on their taxes, take a peek at the answers before the test, slip the expensive bracelet inside their handbag, cheat on their spouse, clean out the cash register, take home the new television set. But fear is a great crime stopper. I suspect that many guys who commit date rape don't have any of that fear.

When William Kennedy Smith was accused some years ago of raping a young woman at the Kennedy compound, we started to hear stories about other women he had allegedly forced himself upon. In other words, he had come to believe that there would be no consequences to his actions—he'd get away with it. When Mike Tyson was convicted of raping a beauty pageant contestant, we heard tales of his forcing himself on others in the past and of his handlers' covering up the incidents with stacks of cash. Mike soon learned he could do whatever he wanted to whomever he wanted.

If there was anything remarkable about the high school boys in Glen Ridge, New Jersey, who were accused of sexually assaulting a mentally challenged young woman a few years ago, it was not remorse or sorrow but the fact that they thought they'd get away with it. In many of these cases, particularly when the guys are popular and well-known and the women aren't, many people rush to the defense of the accused and attack the victims. I remember being quite disturbed by all the prominent and not-so-prominent African-Americans who rushed to Tyson's defense after the rape accusation, as if this brutish man with a history of abusing women wasn't capable of such an act.

For the rest of us brothers, what stops us from taking a woman against her will is a basic respect for the opposite sex and the knowledge that we will have to look her in the face the next day. Seeing our mother or our sister or our cousin when we look in that woman's face should be enough to halt us dead in our tracks—and if it's not, we have a serious problem.

And it shouldn't even be necessary to say this, but I'll say it anyway: In the small, close-knit black community in most environments—from college campuses to the workplace—once you get accused of being a rapist, you're going to have a challenging time getting another date.

Booty Calls

From a Sistah

Comedian/actor Bill Bellamy was the first one to put a name to it. Had this hilarious sketch he presented back in the early '90s on that crazy show *Def Comedy Jam*—talking about how wanna-be beauty queen Desiree Washington, the young woman who brought down boxer Mike Tyson on rape charges, should have known what brute boy wanted when he invited her back up to his hotel room at two o'clock in the morning.

It happens, he insisted, all the time; the brother, looking for a little lovin' without all the other wining and dining, avoids calling his woman to make a "date" until he knows full well it's too late to do anything else but knock boots. He flips through his humongous Rolodex, its pages so expansive they could cool a 400-pound man in 110-degree heat, searching for the perfect person to strike: someone who doesn't have kids, a husband, whom he doesn't owe money to. Finally, he finds *her* number and calls. "Hey, girl, what you doing?" he asks, all smooth. "Why don't you come over?"

4. Step into the kitchen and whip me together a quick snack.

5. Serve the snack to me in bed.

6. Lick every inch of my body—twice.

7. Give me a sensual full-body massage.

8. Go downtown once more to make sure my toes are fully curled.

9. Let's get our thighs to slappin' for at least a half hour.

10. Give me eminent domain over the remote control.

Lord, haven't we all been through one of those? Lord, haven't we all been dumb enough to get in the shower, then the car, then his bed in the middle of the night? Lord, haven't we all felt like complete idiots when we didn't hear from him until he was ready to take a romp in the sack again, weeks after the last middle-of-the-night call—the booty call? (Of course, even in Bellamy's joke, the sistah gets the high five; even though she ends up ringing his doorbell, she shows up with her girlfriend—which means that ain't nothing happening but talking up in that house on that night.)

As far as I can recall, Bellamy's joke "Booty Call" was the first time that anyone had given a name to the long-standing practice of calling a woman in the middle of the night for sex. Or perhaps it was some man thing made up in the locker room world of guy talk that we women weren't privy to.

But we were quite familiar with the process—some of us are still all too familiar with it. We meet him, get asked out on a few dates, have a good time, think all is just peachy keen, swell on the dating front. We might even catch some feelings for boyfriend, call the girls, and tell them we might have found the one. "Yeah, chile—we went to the museum and the opera and the Patti LaBelle concert, and the other week he sent me flowers."

She's all happy for us—wants to throw a "my girlfriend done got a man" party with all the girls. Then a few weeks later, the girl-friend conversation turns into something else—takes on a whole 'nother tone. She goes, "Well, I know he sent you flowers last month and took you to see Patti, but what you mean you haven't really seen him lately?"

"Well," girlfriend says, low and pathetic-like. "He did come over a few times last week, but he was working late, so he didn't get here until late. And he had to get into work early, so he left early."

"Early—like in, after you guys had sex early?" sistergirl asks.

After a brief moment of silence—and with an obvious embar-rassment tinging her voice—girlfriend says simply, "Yeah, girl. Just got up and left."

Girlfriend has no idea why it's happening. There was no indi-cation that she fell out of his favor—no warning that the flowers and the concerts and the general respect for her womanhood would take a backseat to late-night phone calls, midnight drop-bys and 2:00 A.M. good-byes. He never once worked his mouth to say,

"I don't want to see you anymore, but I'll happily bone you until I tire of you and move on."

You guys never do.

You simply start mistreating her and trampling on her feelings. Then, before she can really get a grasp of what's happening, you guys are gone.

If I've seen it happen once, I've seen it happen a million times. And no matter how much we protest, you all continue to do it. So what's up with that?

How do women get put into the "booty-call" category—and what's the reasoning behind it?

From a Brother

Most men probably decide within the first thirty minutes of meeting a woman whether she's going to be filed under "booty call." It usually comes down to this: Would I want my mother or my sisters or my boys to see me with this woman? Women constantly harangue us for not caring about personality, but this is where personality, class, and style come into play.

Sometimes our judgment might be instantaneous, based upon such superficial factors as the way the woman is dressed or the manner in which she expresses herself. If she's squeezed into spandex from head to toe, her fingernails are six inches long and covered in palm trees and rhinestones, she has on enough gold to make Master P jealous, and she is spending more time looking at our car than at us, we are certain of one thing: She damn sure ain't gonna be meetin' Mama. But she still may be fine enough and intriguing enough for us to want to spend some intimate time with her. We just don't want anyone else to know about it.

That's not to say that all ghetto girls are automatically booty-call material or that the more refined siddity sistahs are long-term relationship material. For instance, after spending time with one of these refined sistahs we might discover she's as interesting as watching water freeze. An entire evening or a months-long relationship with her would be torture. We'd rather read the *Encyclopaedia Britannica* from A to Z. But a few hours at a time one or two nights a week in the morning's wee hours, when all you have to hear her say is "more" or "harder," might be quite doable.

Sometimes there may be a little elitism that goes into our calculations, i.e., we might decide that this or that woman isn't "good enough" to be our girlfriend or mate. On its face, that may sound harsh or unfeeling, but I believe it's the same kind of calculation most of us—men *and* women—make when we meet new people. However, the difference between men and women is that if the woman is pretty or sexy enough, we sometimes may still pursue a superficial, physical relationship even if the sound of her voice makes our skin crawl. We'll just show up as late as possible and leave as soon as we can without voiding any future visits. Perhaps the sound of her moans is a bit more bearable than her actual voice.

Though we decide quite early whether we consider a woman a booty call, women actually have a lot of control over our likelihood of making this determination. There are many women whose manner of flirting with a guy is overtly sexual and suggestive—within the first ten minutes she has already let him know that she might be available to him for use as a sexual object. She does this by her words, body language, touch. In many cases, this is a woman whom the brother might have found classy and interesting, but that's all tossed aside once he hears what she's putting on the menu. Right away, this dude is going to start thinking about feeding his organ, not his mind. The thoughts that run through his noggin are: Do I have any time right now to "do" her? Where could we go? Is anybody watching us? I wonder if her butt is as big as it looks in those tight pants?

If this same brother met this same woman and, while she clearly gave him the impression she was attracted to him, she seemed like a fun, vivacious, well-mannered, and thoughtful woman, his initial thoughts would be: How can I see her again? What should I say next? Does she have a boyfriend? Does anyone see me talking to this lovely lady? I wonder if her butt is as big as it looks in those tight pants?

When a woman starts the encounter off on a sexual note, we're quickly going to consider it a sexual relationship. From that day forward, when we think of her we're going to think of sex and wonder when is the next time we're going to get some. If we have to go somewhere with her in public, we're going to try to keep it short and simple so we can get to the bonin' as soon as possible. It would be extremely difficult for this woman to reverse her course and try to get us to take her more seriously—for instance, to close her legs and insist that we start spending quality time together. After already getting the good stuff, we'll probably consider this new act flaky and not worth the effort. So we'll just keep on walking.

Let me also say this: Booty calls are a whole lot of fun. There's something purely erotic about them—maybe having something to do with the fact that the whole reason for the get-together is to bone. For dudes, there is a simplicity to the booty call. No wining, no dining, no expensive gifts, not even a whole lot of conversation. Just booty.

Do women ever make booty calls?

From a Sistah

Women are not strangers to the booty call—and some of us are even prone to dialing up some numbers, too.

But it's more likely that she will accept a booty call than make one—or at least take great pains to make it look like she wasn't calling you at 2:00 A.M. for sex.

Let's be real, here: How many women do you know who are likely to work up enough nerve to say "hi" to you the first time your eyes meet or invite you out on a date first or initiate your first sexual romp? You can probably count them on half of your right hand, right?

It's because they're waiting for you to make the move. I've said it before, and I know I probably don't really need to say it again, but I'll keep it simple: We are socialized to sit back and wait for you to take the lead.

That means that, even in the instances where we're keeping it real with ourselves and have pretty much acknowledged that the only reason we're talking to each other is for the express purpose of boning, we are not going to initiate anything. We're going to wait for you to call, because, after all, we must maintain some small amount of dignity and at least make it look like you're pursuing us. No woman wants to be a desperado—even if she does realize she's being used.

But there are those sistahs out there who practice the Bill Withers's "just keep on using me, until you use me up" school of thought, who enjoy a good booty call every now and then, and even make some themselves. We're not stupid; we know when we're being used for sex—when we don't see him until 2:00 A.M., he's leaving an hour later, and we don't hear from him for a coupla weeks, at the same exact time.

Y'all ain't slick.

We're just with it.

Because there does come the occasion for some of us in which we're simply tired of sleeping in our bed alone, the cat curled up at the end of the mattress. We get into that serious Marvin Gaye "Sexual Healing" mode, and anything goes—even the 2:00 A.M. phone call.

And in the instances where you don't call, we will call you.

We just won't make it all that obvious.

First of all, the call won't come at 2:00 A.M.; we will have planned it out carefully, so as not to seem sluttish. There is nothing more that can be said at 2:00 A.M. to some boy other than "Come over; let's screw"—or at least that's what we think he'll hear when his phone wakes him out of his sound sleep and we're on the other line talking about "What you doin'?"

You all may think you're slick with that one, but you're not. And we're going to be a little less obvious than that.

We're going to call you at, like, 3:00 P.M., at work or something, and invite you over to dinner really casual-like—like, "Hey—I was in the mood for some seafood and I got enough to cook for two. Why don't you come over for a late dinner?"

And we'll kindly tell you to come over around 9:00 P.M. or so, knowing full well that if we try to get you to come over any earlier, you won't. The 9:00 P.M. thing is good, because you get a half-hour dinner set-up, about forty minutes of eating time, which puts us at a little before 10:30 or so, and then we can either wait for you to make the first move, or, if we're really in need of some, say something suggestive or just straight-up grab you and get to handling our business. We will have gotten what we wanted, and you can now leave and we can get some sleep and have sweet dreams to boot, pretty confident in the fact that you had no clue that that's what we were up to.

Or at least we'll delude ourselves into thinking this.

Surely, you guys know when you're getting a booty call. Y'all are smart like that.

Sometimes, though, we're not too sure what we're getting. There are instances, of course, in which men simply can't take us out at a decent hour or spend a whole lot of time with us during the day.

Tell me: **How do we recognize a booty call—as opposed to a hardworking man who is simply short on time and can't make it over until late?**

From a Brother

If that hardworking man has already been taking you out to dinner and walks in the park and early evening movies, then you're clearly not on the booty-call list. He likes being around you and doesn't mind showing you off to the public. Just because he occasionally calls you late at night and wants to come over doesn't mean it's a booty call—he might really want to see you. Sure, sex may be a part of his plans, but he's not going to book up as soon as the act is completed, and he may even cook you breakfast in the morning.

No, booty calls are something else entirely. Booty calls don't vary—we don't take them out on dates. The call may not always come at the same time—it can be in the middle of the afternoon or the late morning—but the duration of the visit rarely exceeds the number of hours for foreplay, sex, and brief after-sex cuddling (though on occasion the brother may unintentionally fall asleep in your bed). When a woman is on that list, we become as slippery as James Bond to avoid dinners and the movies and strolls in the park with her.

There have been times in my life when I knew that the woman knew that she was on my booty-call list. Once in a while she'd make some noises about us going out together on a date, but she would never push too hard and she'd quickly back off as soon as she heard my stammering and I started to assume the liquid form of the villain in *Terminator II* and slip right out of her hands. These "relationships" would end in one of two ways: She'd get tired of me/I'd get tired of her, or one of us would meet somebody special and suddenly not even remember the other's name. Matter-of-fact, I still seem to have amnesia about the names. The encounters were "easy come, easy go"—pun definitely intended.

There's a simple test to determine whether you're on a brother's booty-call list: If you deny him the good stuff two times in a row during his late-night visits and tell him you just want to talk, and then find yourself X-ing out entire months on your calendar before you get another phone call from him, you might as well change your initials to *B.C.*

When You're Not the Only One

Sex Tip: If you're not the only one and you'd like to be the only one, you must whip something on your partner that he/she isn't going to get anywhere else, that he/she will never forget, and that he/she will quickly decide he/she can't live without.

Buy a book or take a class on erotic massage, buy the oils, light some candles, invite your partner over for a surprise and go to work. Not only is a good massage one of the most sensual of experiences, it has a soothing effect on the mind.

From a Sistah

Yeah, I know I agreed to this.

We met at that summer jazz-in-the-park concert, the one where it should really be called "Weekly Homeboy Booty Troll," and all the ladies, like, know this, but they go there in their best suit and their good shoes and their hair all did-up with a fresh perm, thinking, "I know I'm not going to find my husband here, but it sure would be nice to meet somebody, give him my phone number, and see where it leads."

I saw you peeping at all the other women, checking their forms, smiling up in their faces, making small talk with them before you sidled up next to me. I wasn't going to give you any play at first, but then I decided that you were cute enough, your shoes weren't run-over, your breath didn't stink, and your rap was, well, decent, and you seemed somewhat literate, considering that joke you said was corny as hell. So I said to myself, "Self? Don't give him the number to Rodriguez's Pizzeria—bust out the office digits, 'cause this could get interesting."

> It makes those nagging problems just melt away. And it's incredibly addictive. One of the bonus pleasures is that it's an explosive turn-on for both the receiver *and* the giver. If massage doesn't work, try kidnapping.

And it did.

On the first date, we did the safe thing: went to lunch, shared each other's plate and a few glasses of wine, found out we had some common interests. A nice vibe was established. We gazed, smiling, into each other's eyes as you opened the cab door for me and gingerly kissed me on the cheek. You said you wanted to see me again, and asked if you could call me to arrange another date—this time for a Friday night poetry reading at a local café. "Sure," I said, my stomach whirling from the flutter of butterflies that'd invaded my insides.

We went to the poetry reading and had a good time. We found ourselves at the museum a few days after that, dinner a few days after that, the movies soon after. And we made it pretty clear that this could very well lead to something good.

That's part of the reason why I waited to sleep with you. I wanted to make sure that I really liked you, that having sex with you was an investment in a relationship, not a quick-fix booty call with a man who wasn't worth the time, effort, or a wasted orgasm. I was not looking for a fuck buddy.

That's why I was surprised when, after I finally broke down and gave yo' ass some, that you got up the next morning talkin' all that, "Baby, I like you a lot, but I'm not looking for a committed relationship right now, and I'm going to continue seeing other people and so should you" bull. I was like, "What in the hell is this Negro talking about? Just what the hell have we been doing together all this time that there is some need, all of a sudden, to date other people?"

Now I'm going to assume that it wasn't about my bedroom manners; I don't have any and I could tell from the sweat on your back, the heavy breathing in my neck, and the moans from your throat that you like that. No, this is some other stuff.

I just don't know what other stuff it is.

No woman ever does.

See, we figure that if things were running as smoothly as we thought—that you liked us, we liked you, we hung out a lot, we talked about a possible future together, this has been going on for a while—that we're in this by ourselves. We're not expecting you to pull out your good suit and the only pair of not-run-over shoes you got to journey back to the booty-troll concerts looking for more numbers and women attached to them. And we're certainly not expecting that there was some chick—or a number of chicks—waiting in the wings, getting done by you on the days you weren't with me (damn—where do y'all find the energy anyway?).

For some reason, though, it never quite works out the way we planned—not until it's the one who wants to put a ring on our finger. All others who allow us to apply pretty much establish up front—some do it eventually and others not until they're caught out there—that we're not the only ones, that they have no intention of practicing monogamy.

This, of course, is a problem, as we enter the new millennium with sexually transmitted diseases that not only embarrass, but kill. Ain't nobody looking to bring that crap home because you wanted to spread the pleasure instead of pleasing only one.

We're also thinking that a monogamous relationship means you're investing in us—that there is no one else on your mind when you're with us, and particularly when you're not. It simply heightens the pleasure for us, meets the emotional need we have to share our time, love, and bodies with men who who want us and only us.

Naturally, nonmonogamous relationships are also a problem for us sistahs who don't necessarily want to share a man. There are a lot of us. We're not looking to marry your ass (just yet) but we are at least expecting that our willingness to sleep with you affords us the right to be the only one you're dipping into while you're with us. We don't think it's too much to ask.

Apparently, you all do.

I can't count how many times I or my girlfriends have invested time and energy into some Negro, did everything we were supposed to, acted exactly the way a man expects a good woman to act, pleased him in every way possible, and he's returned the favor by telling us curtly, quickly, succinctly that he wants to bone other people. We don't get brothers' need to sleep with other women—and we certainly don't like it. So what up with that?

What do single guys have against monogamy?

From a Brother

Of course, this is the $10,000 question, the query that weighs on the minds of single sistahs all over America every night when they lay their heads on their pillows. Monogamy. Not the most mellifluous word I've ever heard, but certainly one packed with tons of meaning. How does the word apply to single guys? Single guys are going to explore and taste and experiment as much as they can until something or someone comes along and tells them they can't anymore. It's as simple as that. When the woman issuing the order is so important to them that they can't stand to lose her, then they will be monogamous.

It's curious to observe scientists sift through the animal kingdom looking for evidence of monogamy in other creatures. Some animals are monogamous; some aren't. If the orangutan or the whale stay with one partner throughout their lives but the blue jay and the lion don't, what does that mean for humans? I haven't a clue, but the studies go on. The scientists seem to be laboring so arduously to answer the question of whether humans are naturally monogamous because, judging by our actions, it's kinda hard to tell.

Take, for instance, a poll I saw on America Online, asking visitors whether they had ever cheated on their mates. Of the 45,000 or so respondents (which is a pretty mammoth sample), about half said yes and half said no. What does that mean—are we naturally monogamous or not?

I think I can say this much with certainty: For males, having sex with the same person for the rest of our lives is a voluntary human response, not involuntary. It is not something that feels natural or instinctive. Before you start sucking those teeth and wagging that index finger at me, let me finish. We go through our lives being physically attracted to a whole lot of people besides our partners, but we make a conscious decision at some point to cut off these other impulses, to control them. We decide to put our dick in our pocket and zip it shut—we may reach down from time to time to make sure it's still there, but we don't pull it out. We know our wandering eye, the lust in our hearts, will only get us into a pile of trouble, so we become skilled at sexual restraint. I would imagine, judging by the high numbers who stray, that some are less skilled than others. The more skilled may flirt, they may imagine, they may fantasize, but they force themselves not to touch. Because they know touching will likely cause them to lose a dear partner, effectively tearing a big chunk out of their hearts. They know there are no sexual encounters worth that.

I wish I knew what makes some men so successful with this impulse control. Anybody who could isolate such a hormone or gene and reproduce it in a little pill would quickly become paid enough to buy and sell small countries.

The culprit may be something that all of us, black, white, and brown, male and female, probably need to become more adept at practicing: discipline. Discipline is that period of time—just a matter of seconds, really—between our conscience telling us something and our body processing it and deciding how to respond. Yeah, she got a big butt and an absolutely drop-dead smile and she's grinning up in my face, but I really don't need her phone number, right? I don't need to be picking up the phone and calling her at this moment, do I? I really shouldn't be kissing her good night, should I? She's inviting me inside, but I ought to be on my way home, oughtn't I? The stronger brothers can give an appreciative glance to the big butt and the smile and keep stepping. The weaker brothers know they need to keep stepping, but they don't. The booty pulls them in like a helpless fly caught in Charlotte's web—and Charlotte *was* fine, wasn't she?

Over the years, there are a few observations I've made about this discipline: (1) we get more discipline, more self-control, the older we get; (2) it's the same discipline that serves us so well in all other facets of our lives—the discipline that keeps us inside with our nose in the books when our college buddies are partying their way toward expulsion, the discipline that keeps us bolted to our desks finishing up our work instead of strolling over to accounting and BS-ing with the pretty girl in the tight sweater, the discipline that forces us to stash a portion of our paycheck into the mutual fund account every month so that we'll soon have enough to start our own business.

About the first observation, it's also true that the stakes get higher as we get older. We have more to lose when we screw up—though that thought still doesn't help many of us (see: American presidents, Clinton, Bill, forty-second). When we have a lot to lose, it gets easier to practice discipline. When there's a loving wife at home who has stood by us for years and helped us to prosper, along with several thriving children whose lives would be inalterably damaged if we went running after the hot young thang, it's not as hard keeping our dick in the pocket. But when we're younger and single and still deeply needing to mingle, it's a lot more difficult putting that kind of discipline into play, particularly if there's not nearly as much to lose. A woman we've been dating for a few months might consider our relationship pretty serious, but we're not quite there yet—sure, it'd be unfortunate to throw away a budding relationship, but did you see that other girl's ass?!

By the wording of your question, I'm assuming you don't believe single women have any problems with monogamy. But there's growing scientific evidence that this may not be the case. Scientists, many of them female, are discovering that women may be outfitted with just as much of an inclination to cheat as men. In studying the females of our closest primate cousins, the chimpanzees, scientists focused on the DNA of chimps in the Tai forest of the Ivory Coast and discovered that even though the males tried to bully the females in their group into staying away from all outsiders—scowling, grunting, intimidating, slapping them upside the head—at least half the offspring turned out to be fathered by outside chimps. Miss Chimp was swinging where she wasn't supposed to be, collecting lots of monkey dick. In the animal kingdom, the more partners a female has, the more likely she is to get pregnant.

In her book *Woman: An Intimate Geography*, Pulitzer Prize–winning science writer Natalie Angier reveals controversial data from British researchers showing that human females are more likely to become impregnated from sex with an adulterous lover than sex with their spouse—the reason being that the cervix kindly reaches down and scoops up recently deposited semen when a woman orgasms, and a woman is more likely to orgasm with an adulterous lover. That's some scary stuff—maybe Natalie should have kept that one to herself. All this evidence would indicate that female biology isn't quite so fond of monogamy, either. Perhaps if they weren't in danger of being labeled a ho, women would be just as likely as men to screw around.

What stops women from being more polygamous?

From a Sistah

Well, let's start with the fact that it violates every single rule we've ever been taught about how a lady should conduct herself in a relationship. Then, let's talk about our propensity for faithfulness, the female trait that takes on new meaning when we find someone we like. And let's not forget what folks say about women who sleep around.

You know how we were raised: Boys were allowed to go out into the world and, at age whatever, find themselves not one, not two, but as many little girlfriends as they could find. Everybody thought it was cute that he was a potential playa in the making. Fathers would square off their shoulders, mothers would smile, shake their heads, and say, "Whatcha gonna do?" Then that little boy would go out there, flirt with every little girl, call the cutest ones his girlfriends, beg Mommy to arrange a play date over at her house or at least invite the little hottie to his summer birthday party, then promptly drop her when either (1) Mom said she wasn't cute enough or (2) Dad told him that other little girl with the long pigtails and the pretty pink dress was cuter. Then, next thing you know, Shanda's been drop-kicked for Maya. Until Madison comes along.

All of this happens in, like, a matter of a month, and nobody is bothered by it. In fact, they're encouraging the little boy to do this.

And this continues in adolescence, the preteen years, straight through the teen years and into his fifties if no one bothers to stop him in his tracks.

And it's considered okay by everybody. Because men don't need to settle down. They should be getting their lives together—that perfect job, that perfect ride, that perfect house, that perfect pair of socks, and anything else but the perfect woman—before they settle down with some woman. At least that's what everyone says.

It doesn't work that way with us.

My cousin's six-year-old son recently got a phone call from a female classmate, some little girl who'd caught his eye and readily decided she wanted to date him. (Date, here, is nothing more at that age, really, than walking around telling everyone that's his girl-friend—but it doesn't go any further than him asking his mom for extra money so that he can buy two bags of potato chips, one for him, one for her.) Anyway, the little girl was quickly deemed "fast" by the family because she dared to call the house looking for my cousin's son. Never crossed anyone's mind that she had to have gotten the phone number from the little boy, just that she had the nerve to pick up the phone and call him. At age six. "Little fast ass" was her name that day—and all she did was call one boy.

Had she been the one to initiate the breakup for another little boy—someone deemed more cute in her own mind because, Lord knows, no one else would have encouraged her to drop-kick my lil' cousin for another—she would have been deemed a ho. At age six.

That doesn't change when we get older. I know you remember the two girls in your high school who had the propensity to date more than one guy at a time—the ones with the reputation of life because she was caught out there being interested in one guy too many. She may not have been sleeping with either of them, but everyone else assumed that she was because she had the nerve to not limit her options (and, I'm sure, because the dumb boys she was dating told a locker room full of pubescent, testosterone-infused knuckleheads that they "did" her). That carries through when we get older, because often we black folks travel in small circles, making it easy for people to find out our history or know our business. So any woman who happens to be seeing more than one man is deemed by men to be fast. Ironically, though, they'll try to date her because they think they'll get some from her easier than they think they can from some woman who has a reputation for grabbing on to a guy and holding on like a cowboy on a bucking, wild horse. But the guys won't marry the polygamist; they'll just screw her and move on.

Face it: We were not encouraged to find the perfect job; we were encouraged to find *the man* with the perfect job. We were not encouraged to find the perfect ride. We were encouraged to ride with *the man* with the perfect ride. We were not encouraged to find the perfect house with the perfect hamper full of perfect socks and whatever else there was; we were told we had better find *the man* with the perfect house and be willing to wash anything in his perfect hamper for him, including his perfect socks and anything else there that needed it. "You want to keep him, right?"

Some of us grew up to be more independent-minded than that—had no other choice, really. We were looking around trying to find Mr. Perfect, but he didn't show himself fast enough, so we had to find our own job, our own ride, our own house, and our own damn socks. But our sensibilities remained the same: Find the man—because your life is still incomplete if you don't have the man or the ring, let everyone else tell it. Y'all remember the hell they put Oprah through when, after all those years in the spotlight and all her on-air conversations about Stedman, the ring never manifested itself? It didn't matter that she is the most powerful woman on television, makes, like, a billion dollars a day and changes people's lives, affecting the world. Everybody wanted to know why her man hadn't asked for her hand in marriage.

Now, you know if they're doing that to Oprah, what kind of chance do normal, everyday, average sistahs have?

So we cling; cling to the man that's before us, and try our best to make it work—because we have *got* to get the ring. And a part of making it work with him is concentrating on him, making sure that we give our undivided attention to the man we want to walk us down the aisle. So we stick with him, through all the stupidness, all the nonsense, all the other women, hoping that one of these days he'll come around and recognize there's no one out there better than us. Then, and only then, after we wake the hell up and recognize ain't no hope for that fool, do we drop him—or, in a lot of cases, he drops us—and become committed to the next fool that comes along, figuring that one of these days, one of them is going to work out.

But he won't come if we're playing the field; he will become invisible—unrecognizable to us—if we have other men occupying our mind and invading our thoughts.

So we are faithful.

You all render us no other choice.

It is truly a free woman, I think, who can think like a guy—date a variety of men and decide for herself which one is worthy of her time, love, and attention. She can get over what other people think about her; she knows what she's doing—and if she wants to experience dating, talking, and having sex with more than one man, then that's her prerogative, and nobody else's business if she does.

But this is a rare woman.

And it is a rare man, I think, who would be able to handle the fact that he's not the only one.

If I told you you weren't the only one, how would you take that?

From a Brother

That means you'd be telling me, in effect, that I'm not the only fellow who's been sliding into your bed and a few other places, right? That if I call your house at midnight and you're not home or not answering the phone, you might be getting your booty slapped by some other dude's eager fingers? That if you tell me you can't see me this weekend because you're busy, you might be holed up in some bed-and-breakfast somewhere doing so much bonin' that you can't even remember if it's night or day? That's what you mean, right? Oh. Okay. No big deal. You go on ahead and get your little freak on, Miss She's-Gotta-Have-It, Miss Hot-in-the-Ass Freak Mama, Miss Sword Swallower, Miss I'm-the-Boss's-Favorite-Because-I-Work-Hard-at-My-(Blow)-Job, Miss I-Buy-My-Condoms-by-the-Crate-at-the-Price-Club. I'll just go on about my business. Don't mind me. I'll just go find me some more stuff. Some better stuff. I'll call you again when I need another receptacle.

It may be a little exaggerated, but this captures the essence of our thoughts when we find out that the woman with whom we thought we had started to vibe was actually an equal opportunity employer always open for more applicants. It instantly subverts everything we may have been thinking; she immediately gets assigned to a different category: dick snatcher. She's collecting penises and phone numbers, stealing hearts, romping around with no real regard for what we may be thinking or feeling. She's not someone whose affections should be taken seriously; she's something to occupy the time until the right woman comes along.

That's not to say we won't be hurt by her dalliances. If we truly thought she was partner material, a keeper, then our disappointment and disaffection will be profound when we discover her head is in an entirely different place—or many different places. Initially we may be angry at her, or resentful of her quest for freedom and multiple dicks. We may even curse her name and vow never again to let it cross our lips (or let her lips cross it).

Likely though, once we remember how good the stuff was and how that perky booty made us smile, we'll pick up the phone and call her again. We'll wait for a free weekend, wait for our shot at the honey pot. But as we cross the threshold of her booty den, we will protect our hearts with a ferocity we usually reserve for yelling at the Knicks. This woman will not be presented with the gift of our love: She has proven to us that she won't respect it, doesn't deserve it. It's too dangerous to develop any feelings for her. She might embarrass us; she'll definitely hurt us and go prancing off to swallow another sword.

Certainly there's some ego involved in our reaction to this tollbooth lady, who spends her days and nights opening up the gate to let yet another brother drive through. We don't want anyone to know we're spending substantial time with a woman they might have had themselves—or they might have seen a week ago about to give some to somebody else. That shit is embarrassing as hell, knowing you might be sitting up in the restaurant in the same exact seat that another Negro was occupying the night before, smiling in the same dopey way as he was, about to spend your hard-earned money buying her the same entrée. We have a hard time dealing with that, particularly when we know there are other women out there who will gladly shut down the toll to all drivers except us.

If you need to run around, you need to keep that fact to yourself. Sure, I guess that's inviting dishonesty into our relationship, but how much trust can we have anyway if I know you're out there bonin' other dudes? I'd be wracked with worry, wondering where you were, who you were doing it with, what kind of moves he was laying on you. As I slid downtown to taste the treats, I couldn't help but wonder if I was also tasting some goodies that another man left behind. How could I concentrate on the task if I'm asking myself whether the slight increase in the acidity level is due to the lingering presence of Rahim's sperm? With such thoughts racing through my head, I might have a hard time even rising to the occasion.

With all that being said, there are a few instances where we might welcome the news of your other partners. If we have been trying to get rid of you, for instance, the task will become a whole lot easier if you also have another dick or two in the glass case. We'll know we'd be unlikely to have to deal with late-night crying jags or *Fatal Attraction*–like stalkings—in other words, our bunny rabbit would be safe.

When There's
No Sexual Attraction

From a Sistah

I will never forget the conversation between Celie and Shug in *The Color Purple*—the one in which Celie tells her new best girlfriend that, basically, she can't stand sex with her ol' triflin'-ass husband.

"He climb on top a me and do his business," she said matter-of-factly, like "Hey, I ain't had no good sex, don't know what good sex is, and he damn for sure ain't done nothing to change the fact that I will never experience good sex as long as I'm with his tired behind."

And Shug was like, "Why, Miss Celie, you sound like he going to the toilet on you."

Sex Tip: If your partner doesn't seem to be sexually attracted to you, you must transform yourself into the most sexually adroit creature since Cleopatra, that Egyptian Freak Mama, walked the earth. One of the quickest ways to freaky status is to employ the element of sexual surprise. That means to initiate sexual encounters in places your partner would least expect it—the supermarket, Blockbuster video, the park, the elevator, a moving car, a restaurant, an airplane. We're not talking necessarily a full-fledged, grunting and screaming bone session, but perhaps a quick hand job, or a finger job, or some steamy oral sex. And don't stop after the first time. Do it again and again and again until your partner realizes he/she had the wrong impression about you. Sexual creativity and aggressiveness can do wonders for a person's sexual attractiveness.

If you are the one who isn't sexually attracted to your partner, give him/her a copy of this book with this page turned down at the corner. Then hold your breath.

"That's what it feel like," she retorted, real quicklike.

Um, um, um. I know there were some sistah-girls identifying and testifying when she said that. I mean, we've all had our share of bad lovers—ones who were so clueless about what to do with it that if you had a summons book, you would have written them up on several violations:

Too hard: Thought he was going to push my guts into my throat.

Too quick: Can you say "pree-mie?"

Too slow: "Um, hand me the remote—let me know when we get to the good part."

Too much noise: Like, in the immortal words of *Waiting to Exhale*'s Savannah on Lionel's grunting: "Oh, now I'm a keeper at the damn zoo."

What? No foreplay? Negro, you must be out yo' mind. That right there will get you a ticket straight on up out of here—do not pass go, do not even think about collecting ever again.

No matter what you guys think, we women (well, at least the ones with, er, experience) have come across y'all—the ones sweating and grunting and carrying on on top of us like they're doing something. They bring us about as much pleasure as turbulence on an airplane, or being puked on—or being hit by a Mack truck.

We would rather go without sex for eternity and beyond (well, maybe not beyond) than have to suffer through another night of extremely disappointing sex with you.

Maybe it has something to do with our libidos; clearly, there are many more of us who can go without sex than the lot of you, so I'm assuming that it makes it easier for us to just say "no" rather than put up with another night of pure, unadulterated, uninspired, unsatisfying sex. We know we could stay out of your bed and let our fingers do the walking until we find someone with whom we're willing to be intimate, someone who, we figure, might be able to get the job done.

I mean, who wants to be peed on by the zoo animal every night?

But we've never been under the impression that you guys really cared all that much if it was good or bad, so long as you got yours. May sound insensitive, but we just always figured that as long as she has all the essential parts, it was cool with you. If she has more than the essential parts (read: a body like the "Brick House" woman the Commodores were singing about), then all the better, even if she doesn't have a clue about what she's doing and isn't planning on figuring it out.

Then again, maybe it's unfair for us to assume that you all don't care so long as there's a hole there.

Is it ever not good enough for you guys to pass after the first few encounters?

From a Brother

Sure. This happens all the time. She seems like a nice enough person and she's physically attractive, but in the bedroom there's so little energy and sensuality that we might as well be lying down with one of those rubber dolls. We notice that right away. She can count on another phone call from us when that asteroid wipes out every other woman on the planet—or if we've gone a few months without getting any.

When U.S. Ambassador to France Pamela Harriman died a few years ago and there was widespread speculation that Harriman had some collection of sexual tricks that had allowed her over the years to be attached to so many incredibly rich and powerful men, a friend of hers remarked that it wasn't tricks that was her secret, "just enthusiasm."

Men like to know that they are making love to a responsive, passionate person who will give back enough energy to at least make the encounter interesting, if not mind-blowing. We're not talking necessarily Vanessa Del Rio or Janet Jackme: I don't think most of us expect her to do a back flip onto the bed and bounce us up and down like a trampoline (though that does make for an intriguing image). We just want to see some involvement, a little attentiveness. If she's looking at her watch, filing her nails, sighing and raising her eyebrows at us, chewing on some gum, and watching television—all at the same time—we're not going to be motivated to want to go through it again. Or if she's so stiff that we suspect she might have fallen asleep, we're also unlikely to fall in love.

Don't confuse this with a very male desire to believe we're the best lover she ever had. I'm not talking here about getting our egos stroked by a partner who's baying at the moon from our lovemaking skills. We *do* want to be told that we're good. But I'm talking about the efforts of our partners, not us. It is not a strategic lie from the woman that she's satiated that is most important to us, but rather an indication that she has at least a passing interest in sex and would be inclined to participate in it with us without having a firearm placed at her temple.

I'm also not talking about a woman exhibiting advanced love-making techniques or well-rehearsed technical skills, either. As I have said before, if she's *too* skilled it can make us wonder exactly how much practice she gets in. I'm talking about enthusiasm. Maybe even Harriman-like enthusiasm. Enthusiasm can be shown by a virgin or a fifty-year-old woman, a sexual novice or a pro. Indifference can also come from the same places. It's not necessary to have had a whole lot of sex to demonstrate to a fellow that you enjoy his company, that you appreciate his intimacy. It's the indifference that we tend to run from, those women who act as if sex is some kind of punishment or—worse—those who are doing us a huge favor by letting us put our thingie in them. Once we get any whiff of evidence that she has some sort of charity on her mind or it's just killing her to go along with the program, that's when we get most turned-off.

Though we definitely care what her body looks like, an enthusiastic woman can make up for a lot of physical deficiencies or imperfections. Her flat chest or flat behind suddenly looks a lot bigger and perkier when she demonstrates to us a genuine appreciation for what we're doing. On the other hand, a body beautiful seemingly sculpted by Michelangelo will quickly get stale and boring if it just lies there like a doormat, wishing we'd just get off. Oh, the exasperation that overcomes us when we realize she thinks that being beautiful is enough, that nothing further is expected of her besides looking good. Our disappointment at discovering the body beautiful has no sensuality to go along with that perfection will be quite profound.

We will usually give her the benefit of the doubt. If she seems unmoved and literally unmoving by the encounter, we may conclude that perhaps she's having a bad day—or a bad month. So we'll come back for more, trying harder the next time because we're suspecting that maybe we were to blame. But after two or three times, if we're lying there with sweat pouring off from our exertions and she looks about as spent as she would be after flipping through *Cosmo,* we're rightly going to decide it must not be us. After all, if she had no sexual interest in us and was repelled by the sight or touch of us, she'd probably let us nowhere near her bedroom, right?

On a few occasions in my past, I've sensed that a sexual partner's lack of enthusiasm came from her deep-seated inhibitions, as though for her to do anything more than lie there and look up at me would be approaching mortal sin territory. They even seemed to enjoy sex—or at least they kept coming back for more, which was the only barometer by which I could judge their enjoyment. That they could make a difference in my level of enjoyment apparently never crossed their minds.

In some of these cases, there are issues bubbling just beneath the surface about which we might not be aware. For instance, the woman might be dealing with frigidity arising from rape or sexual abuse or incest or something equally horrible. If that's true, then she needs to share this information with us so we can be sensitive to it. I realize this may be difficult for her in the early stages of a relationship, but this is exactly the sort of baggage that we need to know about if we're going to try to forge a lasting relationship. We might be willing to stick around and help her through it—or we might not—but at least we'll have more of an understanding of where her head is at. It's only fair.

If you're not sexually attracted to him, how much does he need to have going for him for you to give him some?

From a Sistah

If we gave him some, he obviously had something going on. But if he can't get the job done and uses his other successes as an excuse to avoid making it better, he's got to go—no matter what it is he's bringing to the table. At least that's what women who want to be physically, mentally, psychologically, and spiritually satisfied will tell you.

When I was in college, for instance, I had a girlfriend—I'll call her Mona—who was dating this guy I'll call Steve. See, I need to protect their identities because they were both screwed up in the head and the bed, let Mona tell it. Steve, by all accounts, had it going on. He was a graduate student, extremely attractive, intelligent, funny. Had an awesome job, too, at the university he attended—a job that afforded him the finer things in life. Boyfriend had a Mercedes-Benz *and* a house that he paid for with his own money, and he was making all kinds of moves to buy property in Brooklyn and Manhattan. Clearly, he had intentions of making it big, and that was attractive to Mona—and to a whole lot of other girls, too.

But there was a problem. He couldn't screw to save his life. I mean, someone could have been holding a gun to his head and saying, "I'm going to kill your first-, second-, and third-borns, yo' mama, yo' girl, and you, if you don't keep it up for three minutes," and everybody would just have had to die. He was a two-minute brother, Mona explained in one of our girlfriends-chat-about-sex sessions, with equipment that looked and operated like that of a prepubescent boy who'd just stumbled over the fact that he had a penis, could get an erection, and, with absolutely minimal effort, make himself come. Basically, boyfriend had an eenie-weenie-tiny one, and had no idea what to do with it to boot. (Special note: Any woman who tells you size doesn't matter is lying her ass off—unless boyfriend *really* knows how to work it.)

Anyway, Mona told us that he was so bad that she was, like, physically repulsed by the idea of having to sleep with him. And she'd even gently tried to show him what to do, what she liked, where to put it so that it would feel good. It just wasn't computing; a five-year-old would have figured it out before Steve did, no matter which way Mona turned it, tossed it, or taught it. It got so bad she would find excuses for why she just couldn't see him after 7:00 P.M. this week. Girlfriend had so many term papers you would have thought she was studying to be a brain surgeon; but it was actually made-up work to keep Steve away. The only reason she held on for so long was because everybody kept telling her that he was a "catch," nice car, nice house, nice guy, nice future.

Wasn't enough. Because besides being a horrible lover, Steve had attitude of life—freely ran around with other women (none of them, I'll bet, were satisfied—just turned-on by the fact that he had "stuff"), made it clear that he had no intentions of settling down with her, and didn't do much by way of making her happy.

Oh, he got curbed almost immediately after she figured all that out.

No woman is really so desperate to be with a man that she would ignore this. She may tolerate it for a minute, but there would come a point where she just wouldn't be able to handle being sexually unsatisfied all the time. He would have to make it worth her while—and no, I don't mean financially (though there are a few of us who will sacrifice way too much, including a good lay, for the almighty dollar). I mean mentally, spiritually, emotionally.

Too many guys, in our opinion, assume that if they have money and can provide for us the finer things in life, all that other stuff really doesn't matter. As long as he has a nice ride, he doesn't have to talk to us. As long as his money is long, he doesn't have to love God. As long as he's got a title, he doesn't have to show us his feelings or care about ours. As long as he's got a cute face and a nice suit, he doesn't have to satisfy us in the sack.

Wrong.

Our dream man has *all* those things—mental support, spiritual awareness, emotional investment, financial stability, sexual gratification—and is ready to provide them to us willingly. He doesn't have two things going on for him, and then brazenly tout the fact that he can neither provide, nor does he intend to provide, all the other things we want out of a relationship. He recognizes his shortcomings and works to change them.

That's the guy who, if he can't screw, will get the chance. He works to make it better, to make us happy. That attitude extends way further than the bedroom; it applies to everything he does with and for us, from the home that we live in to the conversations that we have to the way he treats our friends. He's an all-around nice guy who is genuinely concerned with making this relationship work. We, in turn, want it to work, and we'll stretch our tolerance level way beyond that which we ever imagined, because he's worth it. That means we'll be willing to work with the eenie, meenie, teenie, weenie penis that he doesn't quite know how to work because he's willing to learn.

I have to stress, though, that we know he's capable of the emotional, spiritual, and psychological support *before* we become too disgusted with the fact that he can't do it. Because it is this man who, with a little direction, will realize what we women want: a man who is able to become an attentive lover. That's what we want, you know: someone who is aware of the other person's needs and is selfless enough to recognize his pitfalls and overcome them strictly to please us. He recognizes that this isn't just about sex for us; it's an emotional thing, as well—and his willingness to learn will be taken as a sign that we've found a good one.

He, of course, will not get too far if we've really not taken the time to get to know each other, we jumped into bed, and he was just horrible. That will far outweigh anything we would learn and love about him in the future. We will not want to see a future with him. We'll simply call our girls, talk about him like a damn dog, lose his number—quick, fast, and in a hurry—and hope like hell he doesn't work his mouth to see if he could have another try.

There will be no opportunity for another try. We will have skipped town long before he thought about it. Trust me.

If a woman can't satisfy you in bed, would you guys leave us? Or would you assume that you could teach us? Do you even want to be bothered?

From a Brother

It depends on how much we value the other parts of her personality—how much potential we see in the overall relationship. I'm not going to say sex isn't a huge part of a relationship, because it is, but we might be able to work with bad sex if she's otherwise a wonderful person whom we suspect we might not be able to live without. We'll keep driving that beautiful, fully equipped Jaguar—even if the engine is so broke down that Rodney King couldn't go from zero to sixty in less than a half hour.

When our wives get pregnant, we see what an intimate yet nonsexual relationship looks like. The lack of intercourse can be frustrating, but we see how important all the other things that bond us together are. We see how much we love and appreciate our women for who they are outside of the bedroom. That's an important discovery for us to make; it's something that we should always carry around with us throughout the rest of the relationship, particularly at times when the sex may have gotten stale or isn't as frequent as we would like.

When we're lukewarm about a woman in the early stages of a relationship—meaning she's okay but she hasn't blown our mind—and then we find out there's nothing at all happening in the bedroom, that fact will easily tip the scales in the direction of losing her phone number.

You can only teach someone who wants to be taught. If she

shows no interest in sex and has zero sensuality, there's not much we can do to teach her enthusiasm. We might try to send her hints that we find her indifference to be unattractive and troubling, with the distant possibility that she might not have even realized she was coming across as indifferent—but I wouldn't hold my breath on that one.

What I suspect is that a woman's interest in sex is closely linked to her feelings about the guy and her interest in the relationship. I have detected a lack of interest or indifference to sex when the woman had similar feelings about me and the entire relationship. In other words, her lack of interest was a symptom of deeper problems that needed to be addressed. If they couldn't be addressed or resolved, inevitably the whole thing came crashing down. And it was the same for me: It was only after I was no longer getting anything out of the relationship that I lost interest in the sex.

Let me add here a quick word about the penis. The penis doesn't lie and the penis rarely allows us to lie. Therefore it is much harder for a man to get away with faking sexual attraction or interest in a woman. Perhaps for a short time the mere fact that she is female, has breasts and a butt, and she's lying before us without any clothes is enough to get the engine charged and the equipment enlarged. But that doesn't last long. If we're not sexually attracted to her and we really don't want to have sex with her, the penis will eventually sing like those new millennium mobsters. No amount of cajoling, threatening, or coaxing will convince the penis to betray the fact that he doesn't really want to go there. Not even a bit of quick and purposeful masturbation—for he will almost *always* respond to our hand—will do the trick because it won't last. As soon as he once again realizes what's being asked of him, he'll rebel.

Now that's not to say that women should believe that every time a man is unable to achieve erection he is physically unattracted to her—after all, there are many mental and physical reasons for impotence that have nothing to do with the woman—but if this has gone on for a while and there's no medical or emotional explanation, perhaps the penis is just stubbornly refusing to lie.

Having Sex vs. Making Love

Sex Tip: If he's reaching for his pants and shoes so quickly after his orgasm that his penis hasn't even gotten soft yet, you just had sex.

If he's still lying there moaning your name and clutching the pillow after you've already grabbed the phone and called up your girl, you made love.

If she's telling you when it's over that it's just too damn hot to cuddle, you just had sex.

If she jumps out of bed and scoots into the kitchen

From a Sistah

For sure, there is a difference for us.

Sex? It's just plain and simple, straight-up bonin'. It's the only way, really, to describe it. There is no emotional attachment, there are no feelings invested, no promises being made—let alone kept—no reassurances that this is going to lead to anything other than, possibly, another night of straight-up bonin'.

And most of us have had it. More than likely with the guy to whom we were sexually attracted—perhaps a coworker or the waiter at that funky restaurant we went to with our girls, or even a guy who started out as a (kinda) friend but was just plain fine and needed to be done—but who shoulda just kept his mouth shut because the

to prepare you a delectable three-course meal (or even a ham sandwich), you made love.

mere sound of his voice made us want to deep-dive off the Empire State Building. He may not have started out as one, but he quickly gets filed under the fuck-buddy category. His purpose in the sack is equal to the duty he performs when he agrees to go to the movies with us when everybody else we know had something to do that night, or when he agrees to go to our girlfriend's wedding or to a company dinner because we just couldn't find anyone else to go with. We make it clear to everyone that he is not our boyfriend. He is introduced as "a friend," but to ourselves and our girls he is better identified as, well, a convenience—a stand-in until the man comes along.

Now, the man? We make love to and with him. It's never, ever, just plain bonin', just straight-up sex with him; it's a roller-coaster ride of ecstacy that we don't ever want to get off. He comes equipped with all the things that we've ever wanted from a man—love, stability, emotions, honesty, trust, compassion, commitment—and all of that seeps from his body and ours every time we make love. We love being with him, look forward to seeing him when we know he's on his way, enjoy every minute when he's with us, miss him every moment he's away. He brings out the best in us and doesn't mind when the worst rears its ugly head, because he's confident that he can make it go away and make us feel better. And we appreciate him for that.

As a result, our sex is uninhibited, free, passionate, unbounded. It's never a routine with him, a snack to hold us over until the meal comes walking in. He is the first, second, third, fourth, and fifth course—dessert, coffee, and an after-dinner mint, too. We want him constantly—and not just to have sex.

He is our boo.

Thing is, too often we think we're making love with the man, and we find out—most of the time too late—that he considers us to be fuck buddies. We thought we had it going on, that everything was going as smooth as smooth could be, that he really cared about us the way that we cared for him—and we find out that he was just sexing us up.

And it's hard on us, because we thought the man was the one.

Perhaps the reason why we get the two confused is because we don't understand how men distinguish between having sex and making love. If we could crawl into his mind and read it, then maybe we could spare the anger and the hurt feelings that come along when the phone calls dry up, he stops coming over, and he is no longer available to carry on what we thought was a committed relationship.

So tell us: When is what you're doing with a woman just sex—as opposed to making love? How do you all distinguish between the two?

From a Brother

Are we talking just semantics here? Otherwise, the difference seems pretty plain: You make love when you're in love. We're no different than women in that respect. Now, if you happen to be one of those people who calls virtually everything that happens in bed between two people "making love," no matter what their feelings are toward each other, than we're just playing word games—"making love" is the same as "having sex" is the same as "knocking boots" is the same as "getting your swerve on." But for argument's sake, let's assume that they mean two different things.

The question then becomes: Does the sex feel any different when we're in love? The answer to that is an unequivocal yes. It feels so different that if the relationship ends, it's hard to go back to just having sex. Once we get used to lobster, frozen fish sticks just don't cut it anymore. They may be filling, but we feel no passion about eating them, no glow from knowing it's a special meal. When we're having sex, our focus is generally on one body part only: our penis. Our mind is minimally involved; friction is the name of this game. When enough is applied to the penis to achieve orgasm, the whole show is over. We might as well pack up the tent and go home, because the acrobatics and the lion taming are done. Of course, it is ideal if the friction is provided by a woman, but if necessary our hand can also get the job done. In fact, we have grown quite accustomed to the work of our hand over the years. A woman might scoff at the challenge of surpassing our hand, but she shouldn't take it too lightly. More than a few women have suffered shameful defeat and been sent on their way.

We might go through our adult lives having sex with different women and occasionally even suspect we might be making love—on those occasions when we don't mind cuddling afterward—then we get zapped. We meet *her*. Everything about her takes our breath away; she's a living embodiment of an angel (before her head gets too big, I should say she's not perfect—just as close as we've ever gotten). We want to spend every waking moment in her presence; when we're sitting at our desks, we're wondering where she is, what she's doing, who she's talking to—we especially wonder about that one. She becomes an occupying force in our brains, seizing control of our villages, putting us on a strict curfew, severely limiting the people who can come and go, ruling with an iron hand. And we relish every minute of it. Just her scent sets us off; we sniff the pillows when she's gone, put her clothes to our face and drink in her essence. And when we hit the bedroom—Oh, Lawdy, have mercy! It's unlike anything we've ever experienced, dripping (sometimes literally) with passion and sensitivity, each time surpassing the last in exploring the upper reaches of dramatic, intense, and heart-stopping intimacy. As we come down from our high, we ask each other if it could ever possibly get better than that—and, amazingly, the next time it does.

Once we've had that, it's real hard to go back to "banging"—one of the many inelegant terms that we so inelegantly apply to having sex. Back to a focus on the penis, rather than involving the full range of senses and emotions; back to the quest for friction (remember that Rae Dawn Chong movie *Quest for Fire*, about those barely evolved prehistoric humans? Well, that's us, desperate for friction), rather than seeking our most intensely sensual experience. For a while, we may be sated by the wonders of difference: the fun of tasting, smelling, encountering as many different women as possible. I'm not going to lie—difference can be quite exciting and satisfying at first. It's like a sexual smorgasbord; we delight in the fact that there are so many different flavors out there, so many different personalities, different sensations. But what usually happens at a smorgasbord? After the first time around the circuit, two things occur: (1) we get overstuffed; and (2) we grow less impressed by the variety of the selections. We discover that many of the dishes don't agree with us; in fact, we find a few of them quite nasty and vow never to try them again. By day two or three on the cruise or at the Caribbean resort, we narrow our picks to the things that we really like. And when we go back for seconds, we go straight to what has emerged as our favorite. So despite the fact that there are perhaps a dozen or more dishes to choose from, we have eyes for only a couple. *Vive la différence* and all that, but pretty soon difference for the sake of difference gets stale. We want to settle down with what we like, the taste we prefer.

When we're in love, we also don't mind appearing weak or vulnerable in front of our lover. Weak and vulnerable is a state that most men would cut off a limb to avoid under most circumstances, but suddenly we're letting down all our guards and protections and allowing her inside. It's a scary position for us, to be that open and exposed. But we have trust; we know she will take care, she'll be gentle and considerate. (The second she betrays us and uses her access to hurt or insult, we might as well turn on the hazard lights because she's driven the relationship into the breakdown lane.) That openness and trust is a perfect state to be in for some fantastic lovemaking: uninhibited, unguarded, open to possibilities. No fear.

Are you more open to experimentation when you're in love with the man? Or are you still afraid of what he'll think?

From a Sistah

What did Phyllis Hyman say in that song? "What you won't do, you do for love."

There isn't a woman on this earth who won't find herself compromising herself, her principles, her beliefs, her customs—and, in some cases, her morals—to please someone with whom she's found herself head over heels in love.

I have a coworker, for instance, who told me the nastiest mess I'd ever heard in my life. A single mom, she recently had a beautiful baby boy whom she found out was born with asthma and a few other respiratory problems. The boy turned into a human snot machine pretty quickly—and for those of you who've been around a baby with a cold for more than two minutes, you know that means Mom is getting more than her fair share of nastiness. Problem is, babies don't know how to blow their noses. You have to do it for them. They have those cute little nose aspirator things—the ones with the rubber piece that fits into the baby's nose, and the blue bubble on the end that, if you squeeze and release it, will pull the mucus out of the baby's nose.

Well, my girl claimed that she just couldn't get her son to sit still for one of those nose aspiration sessions; he would wiggle and cry and scream and whimper, but he would not let her get the snot out of his nose. So what did she do? "What every mother would do in this situation," she said. "I use my mouth." As I struggled not to throw up over my computer, she just kept talking and justifying. "You'll see when you have yours. There is no greater love than a mother's for her child. You'd be surprised what you would do for your baby."

Now, I *know* my child would just have to sit still for the blue bubble, because ain't no way in hell my mouth is going anywhere near the snot in her nose. It's not happening.

Of course, I can say this without having yet had the child who's currently squirming around in my belly.

And a woman who hasn't truly been in love can easily say what she wouldn't do for—or with—a man.

But then, let her look into his eyes as he says "I love you," and watch her melt like putty in the hands of a bad-ass child.

She'll find herself watching him while he's sleep.

She'll find herself staring through the hazy glass where he's showering.

Damn, she'll find herself planting herself in the middle of the floor while he's taking a dump.

You think she won't find herself doing a few other things she swore to herself, her mama, and every last one of her girlfriends she wouldn't dare do?

There are, of course, a few things that she wouldn't compromise on—a few deal breakers. Physical abuse. Drug abuse. Verbal abuse. Cheating. But there are even some women who would go for some of that, if they fell hard enough. Most of the time, though, a smart, intelligent sistah knows that she doesn't have to put up with it. Besides, she would have to think about how she would look if someone found out she let some man beat her butt or talk to her inappropriately or sleep with another woman in her bed. A sistah's got pride, and there's only so much she's going to let a man get away with before she recognizes that her reputation is at stake, too.

But when it comes to sex, she will certainly find herself doing a few things with the man she loves that she wouldn't have dreamed of doing with one of the knuckleheads she was messing around with before she found the one.

The reasons are simple.

When it comes to sex, the knucklehead is just plain laying the pipe; the one is, well, making love. When it comes to doing sexually what she thought was weird, the knucklehead is just plain nasty; the one is simply creative. When it comes to keeping all your freaky secrets on the hush-hush, the knucklehead can't keep his mouth shut; the one wouldn't dare tell anyone his sexual business, because guys don't run around telling other men—not even their boys—what they do in the bed with their woman. They might tell what they did with that freak they don't care anything about, but not their wife or their girlfriend.

And sistahs know this.

Of course, there might be some exceptions to this rule: not every woman is going to be down with every sexual fantasy you've ever concocted in your freaky little mind. But she will, certainly, be more open to it, now that you've earned her affection and, above all else, trust.

Because she'll do for love, what she would not do—only with you.

If our relationship starts out as just sex, does that mean that you'll never make love to me?

From a Brother

There are two categories here: the no-way-in-hells and the it-could-happens. The category in which a woman falls is determined by what happens in bed and also what happens when we're not in bed. If we're not in bed and I sometimes find myself wishing that I were somewhere else, and then when we are in bed I never feel a special spark, an extra intensity that tells me this is different, then you're probably a no-way-in-hell. I will never make love to you. What I'm doing with you is getting that friction.

But then there are the it-could-happens. I like being around you. If I'm not in love with you the first time we have sex, that doesn't necessarily mean I can't fall in love with you in the near future. The thing has potential. Love could happen.

I'm not really a believer in love at first sight. I think two people can be physically drawn to each other at first sight and then after they get to know each other that physical attraction could eventually transform into love. But how can that happen before you ever exchange words with the other person, before you even find out whether the person is two cards short of a full deck or a psychopath in disguise? People who say they fell in love with somebody at first sight probably fell in love at first sight with the person's appearance, which prompted them to pursue a relationship that eventually turned into true love. For them, looking back at the turn of events, they'll describe what happened as "love at first sight" when that's not what happened at all. My point is love may not have blossomed yet between us before we slide into bed for the first time. We might be working at a relationship that looks promising and has potential, but we wouldn't yet describe it as love. The sex may even be awkward and not-so-wonderful at first because we haven't had a chance to adjust to each other's rhythms. With the passage of time, as our feelings for each other deepen and intensify, we start realizing that we're in love. We wake up one day and find that we can't live without each other; this may be the real thing. And by now we're more familiar with each other's bodies and the sex improves to the point where it's truly fantastic. Now we're making love.

One thing I've realized as I've gotten a little older is that the sex act is almost like a dance. In order for it to reach its zenith, the two partners must understand each other well enough to know which buttons to push and how hard to push them. They must be able to anticipate each other's needs and reactions. Until this happens, they will stumble, trip over each other, and sometimes fall on their ass. If he's performing oral sex, he needs to know how hard he can nibble without hurting her, whether she likes for him to use fingers in addition to lips and tongue, when she'd probably want him to move up and slide inside of her. He can't know these things the first few times they do it. Truth be told, it may even take some time for him to get used to her taste—he may not be crazy about it in the beginning. It often takes trial and error to find these things out because most women aren't going to tell us right away; some women never tell us at all. We make our discoveries through experimentation, like the chemist who tries different chemicals in different combinations until he finds the magical formula. It takes some couples longer than others to find their rhythm—but if six or seven months have passed and you're still bumping heads and doing things that cause your partner to yell out in pain ("Owww!" is not the most pleasant sound to hear in the throes of passion), you should be worried.

Returning to your question, if the woman has been assigned to the booty-call category, there's little chance that we're going to fall in love with her, as I've said before. She's a no-way-in-hell. For whatever reason, we've determined that she doesn't have the qualities we're looking for in a partner. So when we come over to see her, what we're doing is having sex. We will always be having sex, no matter how badly she wants it to change. If we don't want to be seen in public with her, the odds are fairly undeniable that we won't be falling in love.

Sex After the Hookup

From a Sistah

Things change after marriage. They just do.

It's nothing sinister, nothing that either partner scribbles into the prenup behind the other's back, nothing she ran to the bathroom at the wedding chapel and plotted out with her girlfriends after you slid the ring on her finger.

It's simply a natural progression, something that comes with age and maturity and time and kids and increased responsibilities and all the other things that accompany a committed relationship.

Guys don't really expect that it's going to happen, though,

because the relationship starts out with all this verve. You're always together, you date practically every day—whether you're accompanying him on an all-out concert-and-three-course-dinner date or a simple stroll through the park on a quiet, sunny Sunday afternoon. If you're not in each other's faces, you're talking on the phone or E-mailing or thinking about each another.

> your partner will likely pick up the cues and initiate the next encounter himself/herself. It'll add serious rocket fuel to a stagnating sex life.

And, good grief, you screw like bunnies.

In the morning, in the afternoon, in the evening. Every night. Every other night. Every night the next week. At his house. At her house. At the hotel. On vacation. In the bathroom of your favorite restaurant. In the bathroom of her favorite restaurant. Behind the bushes in that special place in Central Park. In the car. At the beach. Just anywhere and everywhere, at any time of the day or night.

It's what young, excited lovers do.

It's a part of relationship building, a part of getting to know each other. There is conversation, there is trust building, there is honesty, there is faithfulness, there is commitment, there is a budding love.

And that lasts through the honeymoon, and a few months after that.

Then you go back to your job, and she gets back to hers, and life between you settles like an old house. There are creaks in it. You find out a few things about her that you don't necessarily like, and she certainly finds her share of things about you that she has to get over because she did, after all, pledge for better or for worse or something akin to that. The jobs get more taxing, the stresses more apparent. The ugliness rears its head and you realize not that she's changing, but that this is a part of who she is. And she realizes the same things about you.

And, of course, the sex changes.

In the beginning, you two spend a whole lot of time making love before the hookup because you made the time. It's not like you all had anything else to do, what with sitting up in the apartment, alone, eating popcorn and watching old *Benson* reruns on BET. And you two were trying your best to please each other, to sop each other up like biscuits do gravy.

Today she's trying to get the gravy out of your shirt before you come home and find out Junior was playing in your clothes again, and she has to get it done in the next five minutes, before the kids kill each other. You're coming home a little later now, because the overtime is good and it will help pay for that private school you want to put the lil' miss in.

Or maybe you don't have kids. Perhaps you two are leading, basically, the same lives you led before you got hitched, just that you're in the same house now. And there's simply no need to have sex every night because, dammit, after a while, your private parts just need a damn rest.

Basically, things change.

Sex included.

It's no slight to you—no grand conspiracy that we women concocted to get you down the aisle, then make your lives miserable.

It's just a fact of life: Relationships grow, evolve, settle. And both you and she have to grow, evolve, and settle, too.

But damn if you guys really get that. It's like if she's not having sex with you at forty the same way she was having sex with you at twenty-six she's somehow ruining your life, denying you all the things that she promised you when you two said, "I do."

We don't get that.

If the frequency and way we have sex changes after we get committed or married, will I lose you to another?

From a Brother

If there's such a drastic change in the frequency that it dwindles down to virtually nothing, never, zilch—moths fly out when you open up your legs—then our relationship is skating along on paper-thin ice. If our pee-pees are still working but growing rust, there's a big-time problem. Eventually, I probably will go elsewhere for sex if nothing is done to improve the state of our union. I may not be happy about this, but just because our relationship breaks down doesn't mean my sexual desires break down along with it.

I've always felt that this is why it's so dangerous for women to use sex as a weapon. They get angry at their man about his lack of support, or his lack of sensitivity, or his lack of ambition, or just his overall lack, and decide the proper response is to deny him sex until he shapes up. So the weeks turn into months and the brother is starting to get so horny he could eat a horse. After a while, he may conclude that his partner is giving him license to seek sex elsewhere. Instead of poetic or dramatic license, call it bonin' license. Clutching his bonin' license, he might run after the closest thing with breasts under the misguided notion that he is allowed because his partner isn't giving him any. And naturally all kinds of troubles ensue.

Mostly, I think we males tend to be reasonable people. When our wives are pregnant, for instance, we expect that we won't be getting any for quite a while. In fact, this pregnancy drought is a well-worn joke among men. When we know a buddy's woman is with child, we kiddingly start pointing out good porn shops to the brother or buy him a frequent flyer membership at the local strip joint. We know that over time the sex will not be as frequent as it was in the early days of our courtship. Life, children, stress, jobs, and time all seep into the fabric of our days and start tearing our sex life apart at the seams. We expect a few small tears, little holes, here and there. But when the thing completely unravels and busts apart, we start to worry. And it's incumbent upon both parties to rescue the sex life before it gets to that point. There are libraries full of books, not to mention Yellow Pages full of marriage counselors, to help couples put the sizzle back in their sex. The children and the stress are not enough of an excuse to explain a busted, disappearing sex life.

The little attitudes we might develop occasionally when we want some and you're not in the mood should not be confused with the major disgust that will chase a guy into the arms of another woman. If it's coming on a fairly regular basis—once or twice a week—we may not be overjoyed with our sex life but that's not enough of a drought to cause us to stray. I'm not saying a man who's having sex with his partner once or twice a week isn't going to have any affairs; I'm suggesting that a lack of sex is not likely going to be the reason for it.

Would bad sex or no sex cause a woman to stray?

From a Sistah

These days, maybe. There's certainly more chance of it happening today—what with the increased independence of women in the workplace, in society, and, ultimately, in the pocketbook. Basically, she doesn't have to put up with what she doesn't want to, and she has the power, ability, and cojones *to do what she pleases, including walk away from you—particularly if you're not taking care of business. But usually, it'll take more than bad sex or no sex to drive her into the arms of another; one of those exclusively isn't going to be a reason for a woman to creep on the man with whom she promised to grow old.*

First of all, sex hardly gets bad after marriage. It may not be as frequent as it was before—perhaps not as creative as it was when you two were more able to bend those limbs in different directions without having to grab for the Ben Gay. But bad? Like he can't get it up or he doesn't know how to use it anymore, absent, like a disease or condition that has disabled him in the groin area? I don't think so. If you couldn't screw, it was obvious to her before she decided to marry you—and she long ago decided that she would rather have you and the infrequent orgasm than not have you.

But if there is no sex to be had in her marriage—ol' boy has gone from being amorous every night to going to bed two hours before her just so that he doesn't have to pull it out and use it (with her, at least)—then that's pretty much an indication that there's something wrong. Usually, she will assume that there is someone else, some woman who is satisfying her man to the point where he can come home and not be sexually attracted to his wife. Clearly things have changed between them and the love, honesty, and trust is eroding.

That, dear, will be the reason she either strays or books up. All the things that we look for in a man—the love, the emotions, the honesty, the trust, the stability of commitment—have to be present, and if one of them erodes, it's that which will turn her heart inside out. To her, the sex is a symptom, not the actual problem.

There is a huge difference.

Now, add that to the fact that today's women don't *have* to stick around, and you can basically understand how much easier it is today for sistahs to leave a sexually and emotionally unsatisfying relationship. Years ago, women didn't really have that choice. They met a nice young fellow, dated him, like, three times (under the close supervision of some grown folks), said yes when he asked her to marry him, moved to where he said they were going to move, bore his babies, cooked his dinner, made sure he was the man, and accepted it if he wasn't acting right because, you know, she had to think about the children and keeping the family together, by any means necessary. And it just wasn't easy to leave a man, because he was the one financially responsible for holding the family together— and, usually, the only one who could get a job that paid enough to keep the bills (kinda) paid and food (kinda) on the table. Sistahs may have had a job somewhere, but it just wasn't the same as having a man in the house. It's the way her mother did it, and her mother and her mother before that.

But today, it's just not that simple.

Sistahs are walking into marriages having earned their degrees, having gotten their careers together, having gotten their titles and their apartments and condos and houses and cars, and, quite frankly, more than able to take care of themselves. That doesn't mean they don't need men; it's just that they can do fine financially with or without one. That means that they don't have to stay in a loveless relationship, one in which Daddy is going to leave her sitting home with the kids while he's either running around or denying her the emotional stability she needs in order to stay with him. She can simply pack up the kids and move on. It won't be easy, but today it's certainly more possible.

Do you guys ever get tired of sex?

From a Brother

Are you kidding? That's like asking Michael Jordan if he ever got tired of winning championships, like asking Mark McGwire if he ever gets tired of hitting home runs, like asking us if we ever get tired of breathing. The answer? No.

I'm not saying that our performance in the sack is always the equivalent of a Mark McGwire moon shot in terms of artistry and visual gratification—you know, quite a few of us have never even heard of the *Kama Sutra*—but I *am* saying sex can be that magnificent to us. You may have noticed that we will go to great lengths to get some. These blind quests are not something about which we would beam with pride, but they do provide a handy barometer to gauge the importance of the sex act.

Sex with the same person in the same place at the same time

week after week and year after year *can* get boring. That doesn't mean we stop wanting it, but these sexual ruts can lead some guys to stray outside of the relationship for some sexual excitement, because there aren't many things as exciting as new sex with a new person. The anticipation of that new touch and that new smell and that new taste can definitely make the heart beat faster. But often the sex act itself with a new person isn't quite as fulfilling as the anticipation would have you believe. It's often passionless and awkward. And once we have done it a few times, it's not new anymore. So those of us addicted to new stuff have to move on, in search of some newer new. After a while, without real passion and real feelings behind the act, even new gets old and boring. For those of us who have come to that realization, it's much more gratifying to focus our efforts on the woman with whom we do have the passion and real feelings. We work hard to keep the sex interesting. We use some creativity—pressing up behind you at that cocktail party (when we know that free-flowing wine has likely loosened your inhibitions) and pulling you out on the terrace or in the guest bedroom when nobody's looking. We use some fantasy—knocking on the front door with a plunger in hand, pretending to be the plumber, and asking if your pipes need some unclogging or asking you to come to our office after our secretary goes home and placing your behind up on our desk so that we can partake in a juicy, aromatic feast. And we don't worry about all the new stuff that we're missing because the search for new in the end will only leave us empty and unsatisfied.

On rare occasions, we might run into a woman who likes sex more than we do and wants to have sex a lot more than we do.

Though we may try to keep up with her, inevitably we run into the limitations that come with our equipment. Unlike the Energizer Bunny, we can't keep going and going and going. We need rest, regrouping time. And it gets sore. The day after an extra-inning sex bout, we're probably not going to be primed and eager to go again. Oh, we might be able to summon up the, uh, equipment on a few occasions after spending the previous day wearing out the mattress, but soon we're gonna need a rest. I know that women can get sore as well, but it's still not necessary for you to *rise* to the occasion to satisfy your partner.

I spotted a heartening statistic recently in *USA Today*. The newspaper reported the results of a survey conducted by the MacArthur Foundation, which found that there are quite a few older adults out there having sex on a regular basis. Among adults who are married or cohabitating, 82.5 percent of the men and 73.8 percent of the women age sixty to sixty-nine had had sex in the past six months, while 71.6 percent of the men and 54.8 percent of the women age seventy to seventy-four had had sex in the past six months. As for regularity, 63 percent of the men and 39 percent of the women age fifty-five to sixty-four report having sex at least two or three times a month. Apparently, not even senior citizens—those of us who have been at it the longest—are getting tired of sex.

Public Displays of Affection: Why Can't You Show Me Some Love?

> **Sex Tip:** Instead of silently holding hands in public and leaving it at that, you can get some juices flowing while in public by whispering things in your partner's ear about what you will do to his/her body when you get back home or get back to the car or get to **any** private or semiprivate place. It'll add an electricity to the hand-holding because the two of you will be sharing confidential, stimulating information about what (or who) is soon to come.

From a Sistah

It is, perhaps, one of the most breathtaking scenes in all of New York—and the true lovers of the city's five boroughs know it's the spot.

It's the Promenade, a beautiful boardwalk overlooking lower Manhattan, nestled in Brooklyn Heights. One with a healthy libido and a real taste for romance starts at the top of one of the neighborhood's tree-lined brownstone blocks, arm-in-arm with a cutie you'd *really* like to lay one on. You walk slowly, talking softly, giggling at each other's corny jokes, breathing in the crisp fall air as the streetlamps light your footsteps. You might even stop for ice cream, and take turns tasting each other's selections.

And when you finally make it to the foot of the Promenade's entrance and you see the twinkling of gleaming city lights just beyond the cozy benches and the lovers and the forming of the stars just above the sunset, you just *know* there is no other place on this earth you'd rather be right now, this moment, than wrapped in the warm embrace of your man.

You try not to pull him over to the railing at the edge of the overlook— you don't want to be fast in the ass or anything—but you pick up your pace just a bit. And you get there, lean over, breathe in the air, then anxiously wait for him to wrap his arms around you. You figure he'll press his body against yours, nestle his nose into your sweet-smelling neck, rub your cheek with his, then gently, slowly, turn your body around, gaze into your eyes, and tongue you down, chile.

And then you snap out of it, because homeboy ain't even thinking about lip lock. Oh, he's standing next to you, but he's looking everywhere but at you—and the thought of kissing you or holding your hand or standing any closer than, say, two feet next to you is pretty much nowhere on his radar, let alone on his "let me romance my lady right" agenda.

And, for goodness' sake, don't even consider initiating a little hug, a little kiss, a little some kind of visible display of affection; boyfriend will undoubtedly act like you're about to impart a serious case of third-grade cooties on him if you remotely try to show him some love, particularly if there are other people within a five-mile radius.

It's like guys think that the antiaffection police—headed by three big, burly, stinky mean guys—are going to march in, throw you down on the sidewalk, pat you down, smack you up, and take your manhood papers away.

All for kissing your woman in public.

And don't let there be a cute woman standing anywhere in the vicinity; we get the feeling you'd rather chop off your bottom lip and toss it in the river rather than kiss us in front of a cutie—as if she's going to somehow, later on in your pitiful life, see you, remember how (un)affectionate you were to your woman, and fall madly in love with you.

Right.

We're figuring that if we're your woman, and we're in a nice, romantic setting, and the mood is right, it doesn't matter where we are or who's watching; you should stand at the ready to shower us with affection. But no. We want you to hold our hand across the restaurant table; you want to hold our hand *under* the table. We want you to gaze in our eyes as the candlelight glows; you want to look at the menu, even after you've ordered. We want a sweet, tender kiss after we toast and taste the wine; you want to slip away for a quickie—at home, of course.

I mean, come on—in all the romance books, in all those Hollywood flicks like *One Fine Day* and *love jones,* the guys don't have a problem being fools for love—in public.

Damn, how can we be down?

What do you all have against holding our hands and kissing us in public?

From a Brother

We don't mind holding your hand or even occasionally kissing you in public when the spirit moves us. It's doing it on demand that we have a problem with. And that demand usually comes when you're trying to send a message to someone else. If I may be so presumptuous, the message is usually: Look what I got; he's mine; stay the hell away.

We're walking down the street and pass by a group of lovely ladies who glance in our direction? I can be sure to feel your fingers wrap around mine. We're at the mall and a beautiful sistah is headed in our direction? You suddenly are overwhelmed by affection for me. So the public displays of affection (PDAs) start feeling like a brand—you might as well take a red-hot iron and sizzle your initials on my ass. I'll moo on cue and we can go on our way.

Of course, these aren't the only situations when you feel affectionate in public, but they're the ones we primarily have a problem with. The two of us are strolling in a lush lovely park at dusk, and a big yellow moon is smiling down on us? We're going to be moved by the beauty of the setting and our joy at having you to share it with, so we'll take your hand and take you in our arms even if people can see us. We'll even do that on the Brooklyn Heights Promenade. In these cases it's all about us, about our feelings for each other, about wanting to show each other how happy we are. The public be damned.

When the hand-holding and the kissing are sought by the woman to show ownership and ease her insecurity, then it's problematic. Nothing worse than an insecure, clingy woman who obsessively needs constant proof of our love for her and wants everybody to see it. That gets tired real fast.

I don't think it's a coincidence that the longer a couple is together, the less they feel the need constantly to demonstrate their feelings with PDAs. Some might sarcastically say that these couples don't feel any affection, that's why they don't show any, but I think in reality it goes back to their security.

At a reading in Atlanta for our last book, when I introduced my parents to the crowd I jokingly said that after forty years of marriage they don't even have to sit in the same row—my dad was sitting in the row behind my mom. Everyone laughed, but they understood my point: My parents love each other, they know they love each other, and they don't need constant reassurance.

In my high school and college years, I can recall quite a few clingy girls who needed almost hourly status updates—Where did they stand? How was our relationship going? Where was *I* going? A natural part of their clinginess was the PDA, the visible proof offered to the world that we were together, I was hers and she was mine and nobody better get in our way. I frequently chafed at these PDAs because the last thing I wanted to tell the world, and particularly the other fine girls in it, was that they should stay away from me. Walking down the street holding hands with someone was too risky—after all, we could break up an hour later, and the ex probably wouldn't give me any documentation, any certificates of relationship breakup, to prove to future targets, uh, I mean girls, that I was now available to them. So the easiest way to avoid all that difficulty was to avoid PDAs. Of course, that thinking was exactly what my girlfriends feared, which is why they needed the PDAs in the first place.

But now that I'm a grown-up and my mate and I both know I'm not going anywhere, I don't have a problem with the PDAs as long as I feel that it's all about us, not somebody else, not sending out messages or signals. Sometimes, however, we're just not in the mood for all that affection. Sometimes we just want to get where we're going. We want to let our arms pump and get one of those good strides going without worrying about synchronizing the arm swing and the march step with somebody else. **In those cases—to borrow a question you have frequently thrown at me in the past—why do you have to take it so damn personal?**

From a Sistah

Because too many of y'all act like the high school and college ignoramuses you described, but way after you've collected the sheepskin.

Come on, admit it: No matter how pretty the girl on your arm, no matter how slamming her body, no matter how intellectually stimulating, no matter what she's got going on for herself, your eyes—at least in the first years of the relationship—are going to roam. It could be that the girl is cute (maybe not as cute as me, but cute nonetheless) or that she has a big behind, or that she was wearing something provocative, or that she was simply smiling all up in your face. The fact of the matter is, you're looking—while you're with me. It may not be an obvious look, but we notice even the slightest hint of interest in your eyes, when you're pretending to check your rearview mirror to make sure the car behind you isn't too close, but we know that you're looking at the big booty girl on the sidewalk we just passed, or when you're pretending to look at the nice suit in the store window, the purple one paired with the orange shirt and the yellow tie, but you're really looking at the pretty salesgirl behind the cash register. Surely you all don't think you're so slick—but then again, you all are known for doing some dumb shit.

There are two problems with this: the first is that you're disrespecting me by lookng at someone else; the second is that you're giving the woman you're looking at the signal that I'm not important to you and that you'd be willing, under another circumstance in a different situation, to give her some play.

So we grab your arm or intertwine our fingers in yours or reach over and whisper in your ear to send some signals. The first one is to her, to let the bitch know you're off-limits. The second is to you, to kindly remind you that you are walking with *me* and you need to remember that, because if I have to break this shit up again, you're going to get cut.

Don't pretend like you don't get it.

Of course, there are instances—a whole lot of them, in fact—in which we're not trying to pull your coattails; sometimes we just want to be affectionate. And when you pull back in those instances, it's taken personally because we feel like you don't want to show us affection. It's sort of like how you guys feel if you're horny and you've got yourself all worked up to get some and then you come in the room and I give you the back and the curt "good night." It makes you feel bad because you wanted some, and I just displayed, in no uncertain terms, that I don't want you.

Well, the same thing applies when we're strolling somewhere romantic or just in the mood to hug you or kiss you or touch you, and you bristle, like we just spit in your mama's eye. It's a rejection—and nobody likes being rejected, particularly when it involves something simple, like holding hands or intertwining arms or getting a little kiss while we eat our ice cream on the bench in a crowded park. We're not trying to prove anything to anybody; we're simply trying to get some love. And if you're not willing to give it to us—hell yeah, we're going to take it personal.

I absolutely agree that as relationships grow older and couples are together longer that they don't find it necessary to throw each other googly eyes and sit on each other's laps in public. I, too, thought it was cool that your mom and dad can find themselves in situations where they are perfectly comfortable sitting in different places, talking to different people and not physically having to be together to prove that they are, indeed, together.

But I've also seen instances in which your mom and dad have held hands, and kissed and looked genuinely affectionate to each other—in public, in front of people they know as well as strangers. And I think that's cool as hell. I want us to be the same way when we're celebrating our fortieth wedding anniversary. The point I'm trying to make here is that even though they're comfortable not being up under each other, that doesn't preclude their public display of affection. Your dad didn't, the times that I saw his hand being grabbed by your mom, pull away in embarrassment.

Now that's a man.

I suspect, though, that your mom knows his limits by now, and wouldn't push her husband past them. Help us understand what the limit is: **How far can we go with public displays of affection before you get turned off and snatch yourself away?**

From a Brother

Tongues are out of the question. Lip meetings are acceptable at times, usually greetings or farewells. A hug is okay if the occasion warrants it, but y'all have to know when to cut it short. Hand-holding is fine under the right circumstances, as long as—as I said above—it's not for someone else's benefit.

Slobbering all over each other while leaning on a car or sitting on a park bench might be okay for teenagers who have no homes they can go to for privacy, but if one of the two parties lives in a house or apartment where they pay the bills, they need to take that stuff inside. Even teenagers aren't crazy about PDAs anymore: I just read a newspaper story that described how teens don't go to lover's lanes now because it's considered goofy and lame and they got working parents and empty houses where they can show all the affection a teenager's soaring passions will allow.

My feeling is, once the public affection has moved into the area of overlong kisses and hugs it's just for show and totally unnecessary. I can't imagine that most women are so overcome with passionate tenderness for their mates in public that they can't wait until they get home to show it. I suppose there are also males out there who try to initiate PDAs with their women for the purpose of sending out a message. If their women are willing to go along with it, I guess it's not for me to condemn. But if their women have the same reaction as I do when I sense that I'm being used to prove a point, then they too need to get a grip.

One more thing: There are the very special circumstances when overly effusive PDAs aren't so horrible at all: when the two parties are exercising their sexual imagination or creativity and experiencing what it might be like to do it in a place where they might be caught. I'm not talking about those drunken spring break or freaknik revelers doing the nasty on the hood of somebody's car in the midst of a hedonistic mob. I'm speaking of those uninhibited couples who are willing to give anything a shot once in a while. If our mates are inviting us to become one of those couples, I'm sure most brothers would be inclined to let the PDAs roll.

Intimacy with Others: When Is It Cheating?

Sex Tip: If you have some suspicions about your partner's relationship with a coworker, it's time to pull on your ratty trench coat and become Columbo. Start showing up unannounced at his/her workplace for lunch. It's at lunchtime when these inappropriate workplace affairs blossom. Show up often enough and you're bound to see something you probably didn't want to see. If there's nothing to see, good for you—and you'll get some great lunch dates out of it.

From a Sistah

I was a ridiculously broke, bored, and lonely little girl in the early '90s, living in Albany, New York, working as a general assignment reporter for the Associated Press. Rent was cheap. Living was easy. Entertainment was rare; finding intelligent black folks with goals and a sense of purpose even rarer. My family and longtime friends lived four hours away, which meant that I was left to depend on my coworkers for companionship. But after seeing them for eight to ten hours a day, five days a week, that quickly grew tired.

I needed friends. Badly. Desperately.

Out of nowhere, God sent me Darren—right on time.

We met in the cafeteria at the newspaper offices of the *Albany-Times Union,* where the Associated Press was located. Fresh out of college, he was working in the paper's advertising department, just across the way from where I toiled every day. But I didn't notice him until I made my way into the lunchroom to get a peanut-butter-and-jelly sandwich (it was all I could afford, y'all). Being that there were all of, like, ten black people in this humongous building—at least two thirds of them based in the mailroom—it was pretty easy to spot him. But I must admit that he was handsome as all hell to boot, so that certainly made him stand out even more. We caught each other's eye at the same time and did what any two black people in a roomful of white folks would do: We said "hi." Right then and there, a friendship was born.

Now, I have to admit, there was a bit of sexual attraction there. (I did say the boy is fine, didn't I?) But he somehow quickly ended up in what comedian Chris Rock termed in his HBO comedy special *Bring the Pain,* the "friendship zone," the place where two people physically attracted to each other go when there's no chance for romance. Neither of us can explain, to this day, how we got there; shit just happens.

At any rate, Darren quickly became my best friend. We'd meet up after work, go to the mall, check out the latest movies together, check up on each other. I'd even met his family, and became fast friends with his father and one of his sisters, who didn't live too far away from one of my then-best girlfriends in Westchester County.

Not once did our lips ever touch. Not once was a romantic

relationship ever broached. Not once was our friendship breached with mentioning of the thing that we knew instinctively we didn't want from each other: sex. Boyfriend never went there—and I was grateful, because it was plain to see that what we had was special and would simply be ruined by anything as complicated as a relationship.

We remained close even after we went our separate ways, he to Washington, D.C., I to New York City. Close, that is, until Nick met him.

Now, I admit, their first meeting was probably a shock—but Nick's reaction to my longtime friend was a bit much. I'd been waiting in Penn Station in Manhattan for my train home, and who happened to be there but Darren. He'd recently moved to a neighborhood not too far from where my husband and I lived, and was just finishing up his first week at Manhattan's the New School, where he was pursuing a master's degree. We rode the train together, which was a welcome relief to me because it was late and I *hated* riding the train alone at night, and I felt safe with Darren there. Darren, of course, being the gentleman that he naturally is, offered to give me a ride home from the train station. But I didn't need one; my honey was picking me up. It was the perfect opportunity, though, to introduce him to Nick, who'd long heard me talk about Darren but had never met him.

Well, what the hell did I do *that* for?

Darren and I strolled up to Nick's car and you would have sworn from the look on my baby's face that he'd just caught me and Darren doin' it or something. I mean, boyfriend just lost it. He barely shook Darren's hand, mumbled a really weak "Yeah, hi," and proceeded to roll his eyes the whole time my friend was trying to hold a conversation with the man I loved. Finally, all three of us gave up; I got into Nick's car, and we went home.

He was stank for the rest of the night—and, if I remember correctly, straight into the next morning.

We didn't talk about it then, but it came up after our second meeting, when I'd invited Darren to come over to our apartment to watch a boxing match with us. I figured, okay, maybe if I set up a nice meeting between the two—one a little more intimate—Nick would see how cool Darren was and stop all this stupidness.

Didn't work.

You could have cut Nick's silence with a knife, it was so thick. He was rude and nasty—downright evil for the two hours my good friend shared with us in our home. And it pissed me off to the highest of pissedivity, because it was clear that Nick was jealous of him.

He had no reason to be, in my eyes. In fact, I found his behavior rather crass and childish. I don't remember, exactly, when I let him know this—but when I did, damn, did shit hit the fan.

My darling, loving husband accused my friend of being sexually attracted to me—of wanting to bone his lovely wife. He hadn't known the boy for longer than two hours—120 minutes during which he displayed the nastiest streak anyone could ever have imagined, despite Darren's efforts to reach out to him as a friend—and here he was, accusing my friend of wanting to sleep with me.

I was appalled. I thought it was the stupidest thing Nick could ever have accused either one of us of. But here he was, saying that a person I'd known for years before I'd even met my husband was just interested in me for sex.

Right.

He was accusing me of what Chris Rock terms the "glass dick" syndrome—the one where a woman keeps a male friend on the side so that she has a spare "dick" just in case her current relationship doesn't work out. "Break open in case of emergency," that crazy-ass Chris said. And brothers—including Nick—nodded furiously in agreement with him. Finally, someone had validated out loud what they'd been arguing from the beginning of time: Guys don't want to be friends with girls, they just want to screw them.

We don't get that. As a matter of fact, we find the whole argument rather insulting, because it insinuates that we women are too stupid to figure out who is truly a friend and who is playing us for the panties. Like we don't know when a guy is coming on to us, or when he's being or saying something inappropriate, or we're just too damn daft to understand that his advances are an insult to the loving relationships we already have. Those kinds of accusations also make us feel like we're not trusted because inherent in the argument the guys make about our guy friends is the idea that we women would be willing to go there with our male friends if pushed.

This, of course, is all the more ridiculous when our men accuse our *longtime* friends of said improprieties, because we're figuring if we wanted to screw them, we would have done it years ago. I mean, what on earth would we get out of bonin' the boy now? Duh. He looks the same way he did when we met him. He more than likely acts the same way as when we decided we wanted to be his friend. We've both pretty much come to the conclusion a long time ago that a friendship is as far as it's going to go—in some cases, years before we even met your little insecure asses. Basically, your accusing us of wanting to bone our longtime male friend is just about tantamount, in our minds, to your thinking we're going to become lesbians so that we can sleep with our good-looking girl-friends.

Negro, please.

Answer this for us, will you? **Can a woman ever be just friends with a guy? Why do you always assume he has ulterior motives?**

From a Brother

As I have said before, the reason we make this assumption is because we have spent our entire lives as guys and around guys. If there's one thing we know and understand, it's guys. We know that it's a rare dude who pursues and nurtures a relationship with a pretty woman without wondering if he's ever going to have a chance at getting to the sweet stuff.

Of course, as we get older and develop real friendships with women of all different ages, many of those friendships will be inno-cent and true—though even then there may often be an element of physical attraction at the core of the friendship. But when we're younger and unmarried or just married and our woman's friend-ships are with men around the same age, I maintain that some of the dudes have ulterior motives.

Our women deny this up and down, with every ounce of pas-sion they can muster, but we remain unconvinced. At a book signing in Atlanta, the room split down the middle between the guys, who believed that guy friends have ulterior motives, and the ladies, who all denied it. Of course, it's in a lady's best interest to deny it: if she admits to sensing that some of her friends do have or have had ulterior motives, then she would have to deem those friendships inappropriate. What was most ironic about the Atlanta discussion was that my wife accused one of my female friends of having ulterior motives and she even dispatched my sister to investigate as a more neutral third party, but when I claimed that I sensed the same thing with some of her friends, I'm denounced as being way off base.

An old college girlfriend once told me that I never made friends with any women to whom I didn't have some sort of physical attraction. I was appalled by her contention and immediately attacked and denied. But then I looked around at my list of female friends, and discovered that she wasn't too far off at the time. After getting married and maturing, however, I realized that those sorts of friendships were not appropriate—they weren't fair to my spouse. And I would expect that my spouse would make the same determination about some of her friendships—but no! Apparently she has never had any inappropriate friendships.

When I read my wife's account of my first meeting with her friend Darren, I was almost disgusted with the rude behavior of this stranger she described as "Nick." But that's because her description of the events bear only a vague resemblance to what actually happened. In fact, it's a little upsetting that in her anecdote my actions are painted negatively while her best friend looks like a cross between Superman and the pope. My reactions are all exaggerated in her account, complete with descriptive and derogatory facial expressions, weak mumblings, and eye rolls. The reader would be excused for forming a mental picture of me as Fred Sanford. She and her buddy were described as "strolling" up to my car outside the train station, but in actuality she was seated next to him in his Jeep, which pulled up alongside mine. Can't I be afforded the truthfulness of a shocked reaction when my woman, who was supposed to be getting off the train, makes a sudden appearance seated in an automobile next to a brother I don't know? And she makes it sound as if I went home and proceeded to accuse this guy of wanting to have sex with her, of being interested in her only for sex. I did no such thing—it wouldn't even have occurred to me to presume to know the *only* reason some guy was interested in her.

As for the evening spent watching the boxing match at our apartment, in the course of describing me as "crass and childish," "rude and nasty—downright evil"—did I leave any out, babe?— she neglected to include the true reason I was upset. Homeboy arrived at the house virtually unannounced—she didn't tell me he was coming until he was practically at our doorstep—and seconds after arriving, he marched into the computer room with Denene, and they stayed in there for more than an hour, yukking it up and having a great time. Darren made a few brief appearances back in the TV room to ask me whether the fight had started yet. When the fight did start, he came in the room and popped a blank tape into my VCR, telling me that he wanted to tape it. The boy didn't even ask me. I was more than a bit taken aback.

I considered the time they spent in the other room and his presumptuousness with the blank tape a bit disrespectful, but my wife doesn't seem able to see this from my perspective. Surely we're entitled to our own perspective, right? Hell, my wife has been known to feel disrespected at the way a perfectly nice female friend of mine whom she has never met greets her when she answers the phone. And that's exactly the point that we're usually trying to make when it comes to our women's male friends: try looking at it from our perspective, or better yet, ask yourself what you would do if I acted the same way with a beautiful woman who was my best friend. Apparently my wife is starting to get amnesia or selective memory about the whole incident: She now claims not even to remember ever going into the computer room, although she stayed in there during much of the fight and left me and Darren on the couch together, sitting in uncomfortable silence. We have picked and fought over these incidents on many occasions in the past and I considered this stuff well behind us, but when I saw the way I was so unfairly portrayed in the opening, I felt that I had to respond.

In fact, Darren and I have since become good friends—I saw that she was correct in describing him as a nice guy and, over time, I've also gotten more secure in my relationship with my wife. So it *is* possible to get past these sorts of disputes; but that trick is a whole lot easier if both parties are mindful of the other person's feelings and at least attempt to see things from the partner's perspective.

Another former girlfriend of mine lost some of her credibility with me on this matter when I stumbled upon an old letter from one of the guys she swore had no sexual interest in her. The "friend" was asking her in the letter when he was going to get "a piece of that fat ass." So even though the letter was a few years old, I knew that this "friend" had had some thoughts on his mind that weren't entirely innocent. I never confronted her about the letter—I guess I wasn't too eager to let her know I had "stumbled" upon some of her old letters (though a letter from a friend shouldn't be off-limits, right?)—but it was always prominent in my mind whenever the "friend" would come around, smiling up in my girl's face.

A guy isn't necessarily going to announce his intentions or ulterior motives to his female friend if he feels that the time isn't right or that she would be appalled. But he can still enjoy a certain intimacy with her talking about his problems, listening to her talk about hers, and maybe even engaging in a little innocent flirting with his female friend. She walks around thinking to herself what a great guy he is—a gentleman—how much she enjoys talking to him, how good he is at listening to her problems, unlike her current boyfriend. Then one day her relationship ends, she calls her good friend, and the next thing she knows her tongue is down his throat: "In case of emergency, break glass . . ."

One way that these friendships form is that the guy makes a few moves to court the woman and for some reason she doesn't respond or she's not interested at the time, so they decide to become friends. I think this has happened to every male on the planet, myself included. So what do we do? We stick around as long as possible, waiting and hoping that she changes her mind or discovers our hidden beauty. She may run through boyfriends like an Olympic sprinter in the meantime, but we hang in there, knowing that patience and persistence may get us the prize. The woman may have become so accustomed to our company that she no longer even remembers—or cares about—our early attempts to woo her. It's ancient history to her. Things have changed now. We're friends.

Yeah, right.

How far does a relationship with the opposite sex have to go before you consider it cheating?

From a Sistah

Simple. Anything you would do with me, your girl, that you're doing with another woman is cheating.

Now, I'm not saying that going to dinner with a female friend is tantamount to my finding you knocking boots on my good silk sheets in the sleigh bed we bought together. That lipstick on the collar, phone numbers in the pocket, late-night phone calls from strange women, receipts for hotels I haven't been to with you—all the obvious stuff that guys do when they're being unfaithful—calls for some Brenda Richie I-will-kick-both-yo'-asses action.

But your practicing other forms of intimacy with other women really gets us pretty upset, because we know what it *could* lead to. Come on—we're women. And, to borrow a line from your analysis, we know how women can be because "we have spent our entire lives as women around women," and we know it's a "rare" chick "who pursues and nurtures a relationship" with a handsome guy "without wondering" if she's "ever going to have a chance at getting to the sweet stuff."

Particularly if he's already involved with another woman.

Oh, it's no secret that there is a contingent of women who are attracted to men who are in committed relationships. There's the woman who is herself looking for a committed relationship (and she isn't really all that concerned about breaking up yours), who will go after taken men because they've already displayed that they're fully capable of settling down. Then there's the chick who gets a kick out of seeing how many relationships she can have with married men— and how much she can get out of them: jewelry, clothes, spending money, rent. And those are in addition to the various hos who want to bust up his relationship with her because they don't think she's good enough for him, and, hey, they figure they are perfect and should have been with him in the first place—they just need to show him the error of his ways.

So one—or several—of them will start paging you and hawking you, talking to you, and leaning on you. She'll tell you about her man problems, her job problems, her family problems, her baby daddy problems, her lack-of-loving problems. She'll ask you to meet her for lunch or an early dinner at a restaurant she picked out—it will be dark and out-of-the-way and have candlelight—and she will implore you not to tell your mate "because she wouldn't understand our relationship." Then she will throw you the puppy-dog eyes, nuzzle her face in your shoulder, and quietly say, "I sure wish I could find a man like you."

Now, up to this point, you may be too oblivious or clueless to get what she's up to, so we won't hold you totally responsible, won't accuse you of cheating just yet. But if you continue this kind of intimate relationship with her—candlelit dinners, walks in the park, telephone calls at all hours of the day and night—and you're doing it behind my back? Then yeah, buddy—you're cheating. And if you're feeling too good, too tingly when you're doing it? You bet your ass you've crossed the line.

See, in my book cheating is when a person carries on a relationship—any kind of relationship, whether it be sexual or not—without his mate's knowledge. If it is truly innocent, then you shouldn't have a problem bringing her around me, right? Or including me in the innocent dinners or letting me know what was said in those innocent late-night phone conversations on the cellular phone. Hell, you wouldn't be having dinner with her or talking with her on the celly in the middle of the night if you weren't hiding something—at least that's what I'm going to think.

It's also cheating if her being around you is upsetting your mate and you refuse to do anything about it. That's right: If I tell you that I don't like the bitch and I think she has designs on you, you should respect me enough as your girl to kick her ass to the curb immediately. If you don't, it means your relationship with her is more than just a friendship, because you are willing to sacrifice what we have built as a man and woman in love to be with her.

Before Nick and I were married but after we were living together, this came up in our relationship. I'm going to call her Karen, because even though I don't like her, I don't want to embarrass her (I'm sweet like that). They were friends before he met me—I don't quite remember for how long. They'd met at work. I got to know her when Nick and I started living together; she had an apartment not too far from where we lived. And she made herself quite comfortable walking around the corner to visit her new neighbors.

At first I didn't mind. She was nice enough, seemed sweet, intelligent. I could see why she and Nick were friends.

It didn't take long, though, for me to become real suspicious of her. It started when the three of us went shopping and she convinced Nick to buy her an answering machine. The whole time we were perusing the electronics store, I kept asking myself, "well . . . she can't buy her own answering machine?" But then, I figured, my honey is generous like that, so I shouldn't get myself worked up.

Then I started noticing her making plans with Nick—plans that didn't necessarily include me. And she started depending on Nick to do things for her, like watch her house and her kids while she was away, that I hadn't even asked him to do—and I was his woman!

I didn't say anything. At first. I simply called my girl Angelou—Nick's sister—and put her on the case. Her mission: to check Karen out, see if she saw the googly eyes this chick was making at my man, or if I was just being way too sensitive.

Sure enough, in just one outing, Angelou saw what I saw: Karen was trying to get my man.

Now, when I brought it up to Nick, I wasn't foul about it—at least I didn't think so. I simply told him that I thought Karen had designs on him, and that I didn't want him talking to her, visiting her, helping her, or doing anything else with her as long as he was with me. Nick thought it irrational at first, but he saw how upset it made me, and he broke off the friendship—or at least slowed it down. (Good move, babes!)

Then we moved to Jersey, and I didn't have to worry about her anymore.

Now, had he said I was crazy and refused to break off the relationship knowing how much it bothered me, I would have considered any form of communication he had with her—whether it was a five-minute phone conversation or an early-evening dinner in SoHo—cheating, because he knew that I thought she had ulterior motives. His staying friends with her would have clearly indicated to me that he was down with her plans.

Ditto for anything he would have done with her that he didn't want me to know about. If her phone number was showing up on his cellular phone bill at odd times of the day and night, then it would have been clear that he didn't want me to know what was being said. If he told me he was going out with one of his boys and his dinner partner was really her—and they went to eat at a restaurant that was sort of out-of-the-way—then it would be obvious he was hiding something. If while I went away for the weekend on a work assignment, she was at my house, watching videos and cooking for him and staying there until all hours of the day and night—things she would never do while I was there—then it's crystal they're up to something.

The Karens of the world will get you in a heap of trouble if you're not careful, so you should keep all of this in mind before you decide to keep that relationship with her. It might cost you yours.

So, how far does a relationship with the opposite sex have to go for you all to consider it cheating?

From a Brother

Well, there's cheating and then there's Cheating. The first kind is slightly vague, and different people might have different definitions. The second kind is clear: bonin' somebody you ain't supposed to. Let's take them one at a time.

Lowercase cheating involves intimacies, connections, sharing with someone outside your relationship in a way that you'd be deathly afraid to reveal to your partner. It's vague and nebulous, but most of us generally know when we've crossed the line. I think there are two tests for this kind of cheating: Would you be willing to tell your partner everything that you do and talk about with the other person? Would you feel comfortable having your partner spend time with the other person? If the answer to one or both of these is no, then you've probably crossed the line.

Married couples or couples in serious relationships rarely talk about this lowercase cheating. We don't set boundaries for our partners or tell our partners what we consider inappropriate intimacy with another person. Our marriage contracts and our societal laws are usually silent in this area. So most of us have to rely on our own moral compasses. For many of us, that's a problem.

I would guess that the place most of these inappropriately intimate friendships are likely to form is in the workplace. Most of us spend more waking hours during the week with our coworkers than with our spouses. Friendships develop. Over time, these friendships become more serious, more intimate. You may find yourself sharing secrets about yourself, some of your deepest thoughts and insecurities, with your coworker friend rather than your spouse. Slowly, the coworker may start to replace your spouse as the person you first turn to for comfort or for confiding. A physical attraction may or may not form, or if it does form it may go unacknowledged, and you and the coworker conclude that as long as you don't act on the physical attraction, everything else is okay. So you continue to get together and have discussions so intimate that afterward you feel like taking a nap. And all along you're thinking, "As long as I don't put his tongue or anything else of his inside my mouth, I'm fine." That's the point where you take the test, when you ask yourself those two questions: Would I tell my husband about our conversations? Would I feel comfortable bringing my friend home for dinner?

The same standard would apply to cybersex—namely, would I allow my partner to sit next to me while I talk to this person on-line? Would my partner approve of the type of intimacy I'm experiencing with this stranger?

What may make all of these friendships even worse is that your spouse or boyfriend may be your number-one topic of conversation. You call yourself seeking a man's opinion, but what you're really doing is allowing your friend into your house or—God forbid—your bedroom and giving him a chance to demonstrate to you how superior a man he is to your own. And you start believing him, measuring your man up against your work buddy and believing that he's coming up short. Of course, you never give your man a chance to defend himself, to hear what your coworker is saying so he can tell you that the boy has no clue what he's talking about. No, the whole dynamic becomes one-sided: you and your friend against your unaware hubby.

This whole setup could continue for quite a while, but if the intimacy intensifies, eventually you'll either end it or end up in bed together. And that brings us to uppercase Cheating.

President Clinton could sit before grand juries and judges and the American people and mince and parse and evade when it came to the question of whether a blow job is cheating, but we all knew what the answer to that question was in our own households: Hell, yeah! Intimate and sexual physical contact with another person is definitely cheating. We all know what intimate sexual contact is: tongue kisses, petting, groping, licking, blow jobs, hand jobs, oral sex, vaginal sex, anal sex, toe sucking. The insertion of any appendages into any orifices would generally be a no-no. Phone sex would be banned, too; there's no touching, but it sure is about as intimate as two people can get.

Still, after those clear definitions, there may be some gray areas here. If you go out to a strip club with your boys and you get a lap dance, I don't think that's cheating. If the stripper pulls out your joint and gives you a hand job, yeah, that's cheating. You go out to a dance club with some friends and start dancing closely—occasional booty-to-groin contact—with someone you just met, that may not be cheating. Y'all go to a table and start feeling each other up, that's cheating.

I once went to the movies with a girlfriend and about a half hour into the film felt the upper thigh of the woman sitting next to me start pressing into my upper thigh. The woman was sitting next to a guy I assumed was her date. I was shocked. This had never happened to me before, and I wasn't sure what to do. Should I immediately tell my girlfriend, who was sitting to my right, or should I move away and pretend it never happened? I chose the second option, but within a few minutes her thigh found mine again! She had followed me! I didn't even know what the woman looked like, but I did nothing about it. I didn't tell my girlfriend, and I didn't tell the woman to move away. I just sat there for the rest of the movie, allowing this woman to press against me, wondering the whole time what in the world she was thinking, why she would take such a risk—was she enjoying herself? After the movie ended, I made a point of avoiding eye contact with her; the only thing I could tell was that she appeared to be a bit older than me. Later, I felt bad about not mentioning the whole incident to my girl, but at that point I didn't know what to say. No matter how the story came out, I would wind up looking bad because I didn't put a stop to it. So I stayed quiet. Although what I did could in no way be considered cheating, I was still reluctant to tell my partner about it.

Many men and women don't know how to get through their day without flirting with someone. It's about as natural to them as eating and breathing. The eye contact, the generous smile, the telling laugh, the casual shoulder or arm touch. But the flirters have to know how far they can go before they've gone too far. If it's ego gratification you seek—that is, the knowledge that the object of your flirtation also finds you attractive—getting a smile or a flattering word in return should be enough. And it would be perfectly acceptable behavior. But you can't take the phone number. Even if you never intend to use it, you have allowed the other person to think he or she made a connection with you that could lead to something else. That's showing disrespect to your partner. That's going too far.

CHAPTER 1

Foreplay

From a Sistah

Ain't nothing worse than a man who thinks his turning off the light is the beginning and the end of foreplay.

That doesn't stop you all from thinking you can get away with it, though.

It's like a sloppy kiss here, a nipple grab there, a rub on the ass, and you're ready to go. And we're like, well damn—how'd we get here?

See, we like foreplay. I swear it's our nature. Just as we like to show emotions—smiling, crying, screaming, whispering—we also like to show affection. That means

Sex Tip: Oh my goodness! The only limits to foreplay are your imagination and all that stuff your mama told you about what them "nasty girls be doin'." Even if you've been together for years, at least once a month you just gotta give it the full-bore, two-act-with-an-intermission, over-the-top foreplay treatment. You know what we're talking about: all that licking, sucking, stroking, and touching that you absolutely treasure but never do enough of. The empty house (or comfortable hotel room) fully stocked with alcohol, chocolate-covered cherries, chocolate syrup, G-string, or freaky lingerie of your choice, Marvin Gaye or Sade or Jodeci on the stereo, mirrors strategically placed, the phone unplugged, plenty of towels within reach, and nothing but time on your hands. You can't let it get stale. You gotta put some elbow grease behind the work. This stuff is important.

we want to hold your hand when we're walking down Broadway, we want to smooch while we're watching that movie rental, we want to snuggle under the blanket while we gaze at the fire.

And we want you to pay attention to every last inch and crevice of our body, from the time we're thinking about making love to the time that we're actually sweating up the sheets.

Perhaps it's in the genes or the physiology—like the rib God took out of Adam and put into Eve was the one that programmed men to want to kiss and caress and touch and rub and all that good stuff.

We can't like that.

See, we women don't think of sex in sexy terms; we think of it in romantic terms. The erect penis doesn't really get us all that excited; it's simply a sign that bonin' is about to occur. But the back of his neck, the way he wears his hair, the way he smells, the padding on his fingers and the way they feel on the backs of our thighs—good Lawdy—now *that* turns us on. All of that is a sign that this is going to be some good stuff going on.

But bone-dry sex? It rarely excites us. As a matter of fact, that's the last page of the book. We want to go through all the pages before we get to the last chapter; the story's just better that way.

And we're definitely looking for all the climaxes in that book before we close it for the evening.

You guys, though—it's like, "I did her. It was good." End of sexual escapade. End of discussion. Touchdown. Game over.

You're satisfied.

We're not.

Actress Troy Beyer, writer and director of the fabulous *Let's Talk About Sex,* an independent film that took an in-depth look at what women are saying when they talk about guys, once told me that "guys don't feel that sex is as important to women as it is to them." Which, of course, poses a serious problem, because that, coupled with our inability to express what we want from men, leads to just plain, boring, unsatisfying sex.

"It's a catch-22 because we don't talk about it with them," she said. "We're afraid to ask them for what we want; we've been led to believe that it's more about men enjoying their experience and we're here to be of service. It's time to challenge that."

"Today, we women," she continued, "want our careers, our families, and—dammit—we want our orgasms."

Indeed.

Of course, if you're skilled, you can make sure you are getting all of those things on your own.

But it's way more fun if we can do this together. It requires a serious change in thinking for you guys, though.

But one senses that you guys don't even think you all have a problem. Shoot—you got yours, what else is there, right?

So, how about it? **What the hell do you all have against foreplay?**

From a Brother

Foreplay is an exciting and necessary part of sex, the appetizer before the entrée. We don't mind it at all. But we do have two problems with it: (1) Do we need an hour of it every time we have sex? (2) When we're in the midst of it and our tongue is snaking its way down your arm or we're caressing your feet or sucking your fingers or licking your ear, could you please give us a clue whether we're Mr. Loverman or just wasting your time?

Surely you've noticed how seriously we attend to the task of foreplay in the early days of our relationship. We put on our hard hat and work gloves, punch the clock, and get down to business, not even thinking about coming up for air until you have screeched and scratched at least the top layer of skin from our backs with your talons. We're thrilled by some good, down-home foreplay just as much as anybody.

We know that the sweet stuff is waiting for us at the end of the foreplay, sitting there and glistening like the pot of gold at the end of the rainbow. It's so enticing and magnetic we need every ounce of willpower we can muster to resist reaching for it the second you walk into the room. (We're at least swift enough to know that would instantly put us on the booty snatching–idiot list.) But we know there are things that must be done—toes that must be curled—before we get to the end of the rainbow.

That's at the beginning, in the early days when we still leave the room to fart. As time passes, however, several things happen: (1) the two of us become increasingly pressed for time when we get to bonin'—either it's late and we have to get some sleep, it's late and we have to get to work, the kids are awake and might hear us, you need to hurry up and finish so you can complete that proposal; (2) if we know we're going to get the sweet stuff no matter how much work we put into the foreplay, we're probably going to start cutting short the foreplay, except for those special occasions when you pull out the candles and that French maid costume that makes our heart race. It's like when we're young and our mother orders us to clean our room before we can go out to play ball: we take a severe short-cut on the cleaning, shoving all the dirty clothes and leftover pizza crusts under the bed so we can get to the fun and games.

Foreplay isn't necessarily as easy as connect the dots, either. It's often one long experiment, and we sometimes feel like a con-fused scientist with barely adequate schooling wondering if our equipment is up to the job. We know we're supposed to be using a lot of tongue and doing a lot of touching and licking, hitting all the obvious erogenous zones—but often we're not getting a whole lot of feedback along the way. Aside from the occasional moan, we don't know if she's about to fall asleep or present us with a plaque as Lover of the Year. And how freaky does she wanna get? If we pull out some chocolate sauce, will she curse us out and call her girls to laugh at our nasty behind? How about the ice cubes, like Spike used in *Do the Right Thing*? Surely our stuff is lame if we're getting lovemaking pointers from Mookie, right?

And then there's the $100,000 bonus question: When do we stop? How do we know when the cake is done and ready to be devoured? It's not like our ladies come with a self-timer that rings when she's done. Some of y'all give us all the prompting we'll ever need— it's pretty hard to misunderstand "Okay, I need you inside of me *now*!"—but others will just lie there and wait for us to pounce, not realizing that we don't really know when to go. So we keep slogging along, all dried-up and out of spit, our back killing us from bending over, not sure if our erection will ever come back—or if she'd be willing to use mouth-to-organ resuscitation—our knees aching, our ass getting cold. Waiting. Stroking. Wondering if this woman is *ever* going to be in the mood, if she appreciates our efforts, if the Knicks managed to come back in the fourth quarter, if I should pull my money out of mutual funds and pour it into Internet stocks.

Are there times when you need a lot more foreplay than at other times—and how can we tell the difference?

From a Sistah

When we're sneaking into the restaurant bathroom for that quickie? Foreplay is not necessary.

When we're meeting up in the airplane bathroom to seal our membership in the Mile-high Club? Foreplay is not necessary.

When we've pulled over onto the side of the highway because bonin' while you're driving would probably cause us to wreck the Beemer? Say it with me: Foreplay is not necessary.

It is in these instances, and others like them, that foreplay can be shelved.

What makes these three things so special that you don't have to work a little harder? The excitement was already there. Something—whether it was suggestive talk, the thrill of getting done somewhere other than the bedroom, or a gush of horny winds blowing in our direction—got us hot and bothered, and we've been pushed to our limits, waiting for the steamy, hot . . . well, you know.

Isn't that what foreplay is? It's not just a lick and suck here, a grab and pull there; it's our chance to build up the intensity of our sexual arousal. That could be accomplished with a simple whisper in the ear, a full-blown, intense head-to-toe body kiss, or even the mere suggestion that we're about to do something really, really naughty. Foreplay, for us, means turning us on.

So, then, if you think about it, there is really no time when foreplay is not necessary. We need to be aroused to get in the mood. And your sticking your penis into our vagina isn't enough, most of the time.

Don't get me wrong, it can be adequate—even pleasurable on occasion—if you're hitting the right spots. But it's just more exciting for us when you take the time to get us in the mood.

Of course, we recognize that hitting it in the car on the side of the highway or in the airplane or in the restaurant is, for most folks, a rarity—if ever even an attainable wet dream. Most of us—too many of us, I'd say—just aren't that daring or are too embarrassed to even suggest it, let alone follow through.

So, most of us are left with all the excitement that can be mustered at the end of the night, after *E.R.* and the local news has gone off and Dave Letterman has read his "Top Ten" list. Though I love Dave to death, he is not going to get me sexually aroused. Which means that you should not expect that you can just roll over and stick it in and expect me to be excited. It doesn't work that way, babes.

You've got to set the mood, honey, or the sex just ain't gonna be right, for us at least.

And that's not fair.

It's simply a bore.

So if you're just as interested in pleasing me as you say you are, you're going to take the time to please me. That means understanding that only dogs like dry bones—and even they wet them up before they get to the good part.

Is there a nice way of telling you that I'm not ready yet for you to stick it in?

From a Brother

There certainly is a nice way to get that message across. If we've stretched you out before us, reached over for the condom, and we have that crazed gleam in our eye that we only get when we're about to sink into Mama's collard greens or get some poontang, that would be a good time for you to spring into action. What you want to do is put something on us that will cause us to stop in our tracks. Actions speak louder than words—and they feel a lot better.

The move you make at that point doesn't have to be overly freaky or dramatic. I'm just talking about something that will make us realize this erotic intensity isn't yet finished building, that not only can we become even more excited, but we can also bring you there with us. Push us back on the bed and bite our nipples. Run into the kitchen and grab some ice cubes and show us what a cold job feels like. Reach into your pocketbook and pull out them Altoids to do your best Monica Lewinsky impersonation. In other words, you slow us down, demonstrate to us that this foreplay thang isn't over yet, make a bold move to provide us with some inspiration, and watch us pick up the ball and run with it. If this happens to us often enough, like maybe three or four times, we will likely get the message that we're hurrying things too much for your taste. We will see just how much you enjoy all the precursors to the act, how creative you can be, how incredible the sex is when the intensity builds to a fever pitch. We will start thinking about interesting things we could try during foreplay, things that will blow your mind and make you cry out our name. Creative foreplay will become an obsession of ours, each time trying to better the last in excitement and freakiness. After a while we may get so bad that you'll find yourself telling us to stop with the preliminaries—"Just go 'head and put it in, please!"

Of course, not all of us will get the message this quickly. We're not all the brightest bulbs on the block, as I'm sure you've noticed by now. For some of us, the message just won't make it through our skulls by watching your actions. We need to be told. We need to hear it said to us, loudly and clearly: "Hey, slow down. I'm not ready yet."

Yeah, our ears will burn, our neck will get hot, we will feel that flush of embarrassment wash over us. We may even lose our erection. (I've always been amazed at how instantaneously we can lose our erections if something embarrassing happens to us. Sometimes it can even happen if we unintentionally do something to cause the woman pain and she cries out: "Oww!") But you can put money on this one fact: We will never forget that moment. It'll stay forever in the backs of our minds, providing us with the kind of inspiration that a spur in the side gives a horse. It sometimes hurts like hell, but it does get our ass moving.

Inhibitions

From a Sistah

I have just been informed by my adorable, doting husband that "there ain't no creature in the world more inhibited than a black woman." He quickly followed that statement up with—assuming a shrieking, whiny voice in mockery of some hypothetical sistah— "Eeeww, that's nasty!"

Made me laugh, had me telling him, "Now you know you wrong!" But my guess is that he's probably—I'm ashamed to admit it—absolutely right.

There is, after all, only so much a black girl is going to do with a guy before she assumes he's out of his natural-born mind for asking her to do *that*. We have, after all, years of our mamas, our grandmamas, and our aunties telling us that all that freaky stuff them boys want you to do is an abomination before God. "Ain't nobody but the devil into all of that—Satan and white girls. That's why those black boys chase after them white girls. They do that kind of stuff, you know," she'd say to us—or, perhaps to her girlfriends, but loud enough that we would get the message without her having to actually say it to us.

Which leads us to grow up believing that sexual proclivities like anal sex, threesomes, blow jobs, S&M—all that erotica stuff—is absolutely, positively, undoubtedly out of the question for us. Do not ask, do not entertain the thought; suggest it, and you will get your feelings hurt.

"Eeeww—that's nasty!" we'll proclaim loudly.

shot? Shock the hell out of your partner. Make him/her grateful to you for decades. And maybe even surprise yourself by enjoying it. But first you gotta relax. Breathe deeply. Don't worry about what your mama or your boys would think. Just worry about your partner. You don't really think your boys (or even your mama) would tell you when they closed the bedroom door and screamed with pleasure during the very same activity them-selves, do you?

Unfortunately, it leads us into being scared of creativity, unwilling to explore beyond the boundaries that were constructed by some mixed-up of notion of what is sexually normal and what is not. Sure, some things are just too hard to, uh, swallow. Like, if my man even remotely suggested that we share our bed with another woman—whether she be a complete stranger or my best friend—

he'd get a little more than his feelings hurt. Ditto for any man who remotely suggested we try just 10 percent of the mess they show on HBO's *Real Sex,* like the fetish balls or the sex camps or the high-priced orgy clubs. I've never done it, never thought about doing it, and ain't considering it anytime soon.

Still, there are things that I—and a lot of the women I know—have missed out on because we were either too scared to try it or thought that, somehow, the spirits of our mamas and aunties would float into the bedroom and knock us upside our heads for even *thinking* about trying it. Like having sex on a moonlit beach, knowing full well all the other tourists can see us getting sand in our booties. Or being really, *really* creative with the peanut butter and jelly. Or doing something as simple as giving him a BJ or letting him pleasure us orally.

Now, that's not to say there aren't any African-American freak mamas out there. Some of us are way more open to the possibility that there's more than one way to, uh, wax a weasel. And some of us more tame ones climb out of that limited box eventually—become more open to the idea that it doesn't always have to be just straight vaginal sex. It takes a long while for us to get there, though—and even when we do, it's usually with someone with whom we can totally trust our bodies—and our secrets. Like a husband. A husband we've been married to for a couple of years. Who doesn't talk much. And doesn't like our mothers enough to tell her his cell phone number, much less what's going on in the bedroom. And values his limbs—remembers how Lorena Bobbit went out when her man disrespected her.

We don't get the idea that men have inhibitions, though. I

mean, it was probably a dude who invented the orgy, a dude who created *Hustler* magazine. It's usually a dude who suggests that he wants to see two women having sex or runs to the lingerie department to buy his girl that really provocative outfit, the one with the latex and buckles and holes in all the places only a guy could think of. But maybe I'm just making a bunch of assumptions about y'all. So how about it? **Do guys ever have inhibitions?**

From a Brother

We certainly do have inhibitions. Everybody has their limits, a line that they'd refuse to cross. We are no different in that respect, but the line is in a different place for each brother.

The world of erotica is so vast that the only limit it really has is the border of the human imagination. I was reminded of that recently when I went to see the Nicolas Cage movie *8mm.* That movie took me on an unexpected trip into the dark, disgusting netherworld of over-the-edge pornography, extreme S&M, and "snuff films," porn flicks in which it appears that someone—usually the woman—is killed during sex. I was so bothered and grossed-out by the images on the screen that the movie stayed with me for days, sending unwanted scenes marching across my mind without provocation. I was clearly watching stuff that was *way* past my limit. Those feminists who claim that all porn is degrading and dangerous to women would have an easy case with the stuff in that movie. But I'd suppose there were people out there who were turned on by the things they saw—not even porn that extreme was too much for them (y'all are some sick individuals, but you probably already know that).

Many guys would be resistant to sex acts that would make them appear to be soft or interested in homosexuality. That's not to say that they wouldn't be turned on by some of this stuff; they just wouldn't allow themselves to indulge for fear that they'd appear to be gay—or for fear that perhaps they'd enjoy it. This kind of attitude is rampant among males in the black community, which isn't exactly the most enlightened group when it comes to homosexuality. Yeah, a lot of us are finally getting to the live-and-let-live state of mind, but many African-Americans are still quite actively discriminating—or worse—against gays, using all kinds of theories ranging from the biblical to black genocide to justify their behavior. (For most of us, the second we stepped foot into elementary school for the first time, we were so thoroughly indoctrinated with a fear of homosexuality and of being accused of it that our reactions are knee-jerk quick as adults when we suspect that we are in any way being linked to homosexual thoughts, actions, or attitudes. Of course, psychologists have a name for that: homophobia.)

All this talk about homosexuality is to explain the origins of one of our biggest inhibitions as men. If you ask us to put on panties or high heels, several parallel thoughts will probably run through our heads:

Does she think I'd like that?

Why does she think I'd like that?

Does she think I'm a homo?

What if I *did* like that?

For most of us, it's just too dangerous to chance it. We don't need that kind of insecurity lurking—if I like to wear an occasional dress, does that mean I secretly want a penis in my mouth, too?

And if we happen to be aware of occasional homosexual urges and are laboring diligently to purge them from our souls, the last thing we're going to want is to put on a dress in front of our woman and let her see that we kinda like it. We don't want her to start having E. Lynn Harris visions, to start imagining that we're living the kind of secret life of the male characters in his books: living with Judy but sleeping with Rudy.

Sometimes, we also hold back because we suspect that revealing some of our wilder sexual desires and fantasies might be too much for our women. We grow up knowing that females already think we're nastier than they are; this feeling stays with us as adults. If we're going to give them more ammunition to think this way about us, we're going to do it reluctantly, sparingly, with much trepidation about what she'll think of us. Many of us may never do it at all, particularly if we think her reaction would be so strong that we'd get our feelings hurt.

We all have our limits. How would it make you feel if we tried to push you beyond one of yours?

From a Sistah

I'm no Vanessa Del Rio—and I sure as hell ain't Janet Jackme. I will never, ever in life do half the stuff Lil' Kim says she would like to do—particularly the fantasy she has that involves her cootchie and the Harlem Boys Choir. And all that yang that Foxy Brown talks in her rap songs is pretty much out of the question for this thirty-one-year-old woman, too. Only a woman can push herself beyond her limits. Anything you do to try to push her past where she's willing to go will be taken as a sign that she needs to haul ass,

*quick, fast, and in a hurry, because you are obviously way too freaky
for her taste.*

There may be a reason for her resistance; it may be morally
against everything she believes in, she may have tried it with someone else and just didn't enjoy it (though you'll never be privy to
that information), she may think she's simply physically incapable
of doing it, or she may think someone's going to find out and use it
against her.

Or she simply may not want to. Ever.

That's not to say that you have to trade in your dream of having
sex with your woman on the fifty-yard line at Giants Stadium at
precisely the stroke of midnight after a home-game win. It's just
that there will be no way you will be able to convince her to put on
cleats and get turf burns on her ass unless she *wants* to do it—and
even that will come only after her curiosity gets the best of her
(read: she's tired of the three positions you guys hit every other
night) *and* you guys have been together long enough for her to trust
that you will keep what you two do on the down-low.

Now, it's hard for me to come out with this, particularly since
my momma may be reading this book right this very minute, but I
recently watched some porn videos. (It was for research for this
book, Mom, I swear!) Anyway, Nick is somewhat of a connoisseur—
can expound the virtues of the Buttman series, can talk about the
enthusiasm of Vanessa Del Rio, the freakiness of Janet Jackme, the
vast difference between a video featuring black characters (way
more interesting to watch, he says) and one featuring white ones
(they just can't move it like we can, he insists).

But he's always respected the fact that I wasn't into them. He'd always known—because I did not hesitate to tell him—that to me, they were altogether embarrassing and sickening—exploitative and overly nasty. I had no interest in watching some grubby-looking man lay up there and let some crackhead looking woman with fake boobs and a weave suck on his penis, then let him ram it inside her while he pulls her hair or flips her around the room for the cameras—and everyone with eyes—to see. Just not my gig.

But I have to admit that as we were writing this book and we started to explore different forms of sensuality and sexuality and talk about things that we've never talked about—even though we've been together for years and are, as far as I'm concerned, quite satisfied sexually—I got more curious. If I was going to write about creativity and talk about inhibitions, I had to figure out just how uninhibited other women were. If I was going to say that porn movies are disgusting, I had best watch one so that I could rest assured that I knew what I was talking about.

So I told Nick I wanted to see one—for, you know, research. He happily strolled off to some hole-in-the-wall video store in East Orange, New Jersey, and picked up two porn movies for his curious wife, then stopped what he was doing to watch them with me. We popped the video into the VCR, propped up the pillows, and settled into our bed—he anxious to see my reaction, I amazed that I was about to watch people do it, with my husband at my side.

You know what? It wasn't that bad. It was just people having sex. In fact, I found it to be quite a bore. There was no plot or subtext, just people screwing. They weren't doing anything any different from what my husband and I have done; in fact, I found myself remembering some of the things we've done together and thinking that those women and men didn't have anything on me and Nick. There was no foreplay, no sweet whispers, no intimacy, no candles, no Hershey's dark chocolate syrup . . . uh, you get my point. It was just straight bonin'—just the physical act. After about twenty minutes, I was ready to pop in the next one. I mean, how long can you possibly sit there and watch couple after couple have oral sex, then hit it from behind, the side, then her on top, then him taking his penis out and going for the "cum shot," in which he sprays his sperm all over her breasts and in her mouth? Yawn.

The second one was a little more interesting, as there was a history behind the Buttman series. Some guy goes around the world with his camera and well-endowed friend, and they seek out women with big butts (well, they are white guys, so the butts are going to be only so big) and figure out a way to con them into having sex with the friend. Then, of course, they got back to the usual fare: oral sex, from behind, on top, cum shot. I fell asleep on it.

And the next morning, I laughed at myself, because all these years I've been afraid to watch them, afraid that they were doing something hellishly freaky in the movies, that I would be embarrassed to watch it, that the moral gods would sweep down into my bedroom, check my VCR, and say, "Yup, she was watching a porn movie—she's officially barred from the good girl club."

The moral of the story? To his credit, Nick never forced me to watch them. I never walked into the living room and found him staring at the TV screen, mesmerized by Buttman's latest adventure. He never forced me into the X-rated section of the local video store. He never told me I was wrong for not wanting to see them. He simply explained to me that he didn't find anything wrong with porn movies and left it at that. No pushing. No cajoling. No guilting.

And I learned something: that though they don't turn me on, I am no longer inhibited when it comes to porn flicks. I mean, I could see how someone *might* get turned on by it, and that's a good thing for that person's sexual gratification—it's not fair for me to judge someone harshly because of what turns them on. Porn and S&M are really no different in terms of turn-ons than stuffed animals, flowers, and candlelit bubble baths, if you think about it with an open mind. And overcoming those inhibitions is what makes sex a mind-blowing trip.

Of course, the beauty of my watching those porn flicks was that I came to my own conclusion it was something that I wanted to do and not something that I did because my man was pressuring me.

There is a huge difference.

We don't get the feeling that you guys are as hard to convince when it comes to doing something that you might have been against doing—until someone, that is, suggested you do it together. We assume that if we suggest it, you guys are down, and that there will be no repercussions for us asking. Is that true? **How would you guys feel if we tried to push you beyond your limits?**

From a Brother

At first we wouldn't feel right at all. We'd be scared; we'd be resentful of you for making us scared; we'd start thinking about why we were scared; we'd be resentful of you for making us think about why we were scared; we'd start to wonder what it might feel like to go along with you; we'd start thinking about how cool it was that we had a freak mama who was interested in trying such out-there freaky things; we'd start wondering if you'd ever done this before with somebody else; we'd think about the last Negro you dumped to go out with us; we'd wonder if he was willing to do it; we'd be resentful of you for asking us to do something you did with him; we'd wonder if he was willing to do it that meant he was a better, stronger, more secure man than we; we'd wonder if we're being too wimpy by being scared, that maybe our fear meant we were homophobic; we'd be resentful of you for making us wonder if we were homophobic and wimpy; we'd remember the things that you agreed to do upon our urging although you were reluctant and afraid at first; we'd think how cool it was that we had a woman who was willing to give it a try even if she was a little scared; we'd become ashamed for questioning your motives and your sexual history; we'd wonder if it'd stay in our bedroom or if you might talk about it with all your girls, meaning their men would soon find out and eventually our homeys would know—but possibly never tell us they know, keeping it to themselves for their amusement when we weren't around; we'd remember that you told us what we did in our bedroom stayed in our bedroom and we'd want to believe you, we'd kinda believe you, we'd have to believe you; we'd decide that it might not be so bad; we'd do it.

It might be helpful to me to know that if I gave in, there'd be a nice prize for me at the end: your agreeing to throw away one of your inhibitions and cross the line with me on something I'd been wanting you to do. So it could become a sort of sexual game, with each of us handing the other a gift-wrapped present that would add more freedom, spontaneity, and intensity to our sex life. That wouldn't be too bad at all. But you should go first—before you pull out that big scary black dildo and aim it at me, I get to pull out the video camera and aim it at you. And you did say this stayed right here in our bedroom, right? We just need to hear you repeat that a few more times. We don't want to seem too paranoid, but maybe you could put it in writing.

Over the years, as our inhibitions stretch a bit, we start to realize that our sexuality is really no one's business but our own and the person we're doing it with. This is a hard concept to grasp in the early years, when it seemed like whatever we did and whoever we did it with immediately became front-page news. Our fears aren't helped by the conversations we sometimes overhear, during which the sistahs thoroughly diss the brothers who are romantically and erotically challenged. If they're slogging that brother's name through the mud, what's to prevent my nervous ass from becoming the subject of next week's meeting?

Creativity: Who's Responsible for Making Sex Sizzle?

Sex Tip: Sometimes it might be difficult to know what constitutes sexual creativity, particularly when your partner is standing over you complaining that you're not creative enough. One suggestion you might try is listening to Lil' Kim CDs for some ideas— but that won't work if you don't know what "drinkin' babies" means. How 'bout this: Think of the nastiest, most outrageous, funkiest, booty-drippin', organ-lickin' sexual act that's ever crossed your mind, then add some whipped cream, a

From a Sistah

The funny thing about it is that you guys act as if you all have a lock on creativity, like we don't know anything beyond the missionary position and you guys were born with the lessons of the *Kama Sutra* tattooed on your brain.

Yeah.

Surely, you all can't seriously believe that we haven't picked up a thang or five here and there. I mean, we can understand you all *wanting* to think we're, like, virginal, and you all are teaching us something new. But the fact remains that as we grow older, and with each intimate relationship we have, we learn things that are likely to turn him on and turn him out, as well as the things that make us feel like we're swinging from the chandelier. Shoot—we might even know how to swing from the chandelier without messing up a single grain of the plaster, and how to fix it if *you* mess up and make it come tumbling down!

Thing is, we don't let you know any of this up front—would rather cut off our left hand and swallow the fingers whole than let you think we're freaks. You all probably know why, but I'm going to make it crystal for you: Just like anything else that has to do with physical attraction, dating, and mating, we sistahs want—and in a lot of cases, need—the brother to take the lead. Mama always told us not to say "hi" to a man unless he says "hi" first. Don't call him first, let him call you. Don't ask him out on a date, wait for him to ask you.

"Sit back and let him be the man, honey—you do remember Eve, don't you?"

Anything outside of that is just plain—well, you know—fast. And we don't want to be perceived as sluts, because we all know

spatula, and uneven parellel bars. If you're still drawing a blank, you should go for the props: Take your mate to a nice hotel, order up a sumptuous room service meal, run a steaming bath, invite your mate to sink into the water, and feed him/her dessert while he/she is allowing the hot water to drain every bit of tension and stress from his/her body. Once you've gotten to that point, it really doesn't matter what happens next—your mate is a mound of quivering jelly in your hands.

that sluts aren't the women men want to keep around. It's no secret that a lot of us want to be kept.

Surely, things aren't going to change behind bedroom doors. In fact, they'll intensify a billion times over. It's of the utmost importance to us that this man standing before us believe we are— hmm, a delicate way to put it—virgins. Or at least that we don't have that much experience.

Men like that.

So how would it look in your eyes if we handled the southern excursion, or the right leg behind the left ear, or the chandelier thing like we'd been on this trip before—over and over again?

Our best guess is, not too good.

So we pretend we've never been behind the wheel and we need direction. A little guidance. "Like this, baby?"

At some point, though, that becomes tiring. We get older, and we think, "Surely, this brother knows he ain't the first. Shoot—I'm gonna get my groove on." Happy is as happy does. Then we throw a lil' sumthin' sumthin' on him, and he gives us the eye— like he's trying to remember if we've ever given him any indication of how many men we've been with and exactly what all we did with them. And before we know it, you all commence to rolling over, not for the new position, but to simply get away from Lil' Miss Freaky. And we know instantly that at the heart of your discontent is your little boy "somebody made it there before me" jealousy.

So, to square things away the next time, we quickly jump back into virgin mode, collect our senses, and hit the missionary. We want, after all, to keep you. We'll just lay back and hope you get a little more creative your damn self so that we can get back to some mind-boggling sex.

Maybe we're simply paranoid, though I doubt that we are. So perhaps you could help us with this one: **How creative can we be before you all decide we're simply freaks who probably had a lot (read: too much) experience with other guys before we got to you?**

From a Brother

We like creativity a whole lot. We just don't like the idea that it's something you have done before, with someone else. We want to believe that we were your muse, the inspiration for your creative spark. So it's all a matter of how the creativity is introduced to us. It can't feel well rehearsed. You can't pull a well-stocked black bag that we've never seen before from underneath the bed. You shouldn't say, "Rodney liked it when I did this." In other words, if you're going to pull out some toys, we need to see the receipt.

We very much enjoy the idea that our lover is free of inhibitions, that she's willing to keep up with us step for step as we explore the boundaries of pleasure. That's exciting as hell. It means that our lovemaking won't ever grow stale, that we won't grow bored with each other as so many couples do. We'll never fully know what to expect when we turn off the lights—or sometimes, when the lights stay on. Our years together will be one long thrilling ride.

Just as with enthusiasm, creativity doesn't have to arise only after years of experimentation and practice. A woman who is a sexual novice can still be down for delving into the world of erotic possibility. So I don't think I'm being unrealistic in asking that we get the creativity without the plain evidence of years of practice.

Our unwillingness to confront your sexual history might sound silly or impractical to some women, further evidence that we must still force our women into the Madonna–whore dichotomy. I can just hear the feminists now, dissecting our head-in-the-sand approach, deconstructing the male desire to evade the image of his woman with another guy. But I think it's more possessiveness than chauvinism or naïveté—the same possessiveness that our women also carry with them. But instead of applying it to our previous sex lives, their possessiveness surfaces when we happen to glance in another woman's direction or linger too long on a sexy video when flipping the channels. The idea of her man sweating Janet Jackson or Vanessa Williams might make some women sweat; for us, it's the picture of our lady having done the same thing with her ex that she does now with us.

And, of course, numbers matter here. How many other dudes were there exactly? It's a question that haunts us, but we probably don't need the answer. An acquaintance of mine who used to play pro football said he became Columbo and checked with every other guy on the team before he married his wife to see if she had any kind of reputation. He went at the task with seriousness, too. And what would he have brought himself besides grief if he got any of the answers he feared? He had already fallen in love with the woman— it was too late to change that. But it was all about his pride, about his ego. He couldn't abide by the possibility that there might be some other fellows out there laughing at his choice of a mate.

As I mentioned before, creativity is a necessity if the relationship is going to stay fresh. Once we find the position we like, the time we like to do it, how many licks it takes to get her going, and how many strokes with how much force we need to push her over the brink, we're going to grow comfortable doing it the way we like to do it. Next thing we know, we've fallen into a sexual rut. It's become old hat. Sure, it may still be good enough to bring both of us to orgasm, but can you say B-O-R-I-N-G? Most couples aren't at the point where they're comfortable telling the other that things have gotten boring. So it remains unsaid—and one night we look up in the throes of our passion and notice that she's yawning. We must make things interesting well before we get to any yawns. That doesn't mean ceiling swings and hot wax every night, but it does mean the missionary position at 11:40 after the evening news two or three times a week is not working. Splurging for a weekend and romping around in a fancy hotel room can have a magical effect on the creative juices—and we might find out we're a lot more limber than we thought as we twist our bodies into a whole range of interesting positions in that nice big Jacuzzi. Or the backseat of the car—that familiar but forgotten friend—may be a great deal more fun than we remember, even when the car is parked in the garage!

Just as it's necessary for us to put effort into all the other aspects of our relationship, sexual creativity should never become a stranger to us.

Is it important for your man to get a high rating on the creativity scale?

From a Sistah

Hell, yeah! Ain't nothing worse than a man who's only got three positions and knows how to do only two of them effectively. It's like

*being in your mother's house, knowing full well that her menu has
never changed—and never will: baked chicken on Sunday, leftovers
on Tuesday, meatloaf and mashed potatoes on Wednesday, fried
chicken on Thursday, fried fish on Friday, potluck on Saturday.*

*After a while, it all tastes the same, and you find yourself won-
dering if you should sneak out and get some Burger King while she's
sleep; something quick and fast—but different—to satisfy your
appetite.*

Not that we would sneak out on you while we're married,
mind you; once we've committed to you, we've pretty much evalu-
ated everything about you, including your sexual prowess, and
have decided that it works well enough for us to continue doing it
for the rest of our lifetimes. That's not to say that we'll accept, after
a while, that your creative juices have run dry; it's simply to say that
if you are our husband, we'll know that it's important either to let
you know that what you're doing has grown stale, or whip some
stuff up ourselves. Leaving our panties at home when we go out to
dinner—and finding a thrilling way to inform our partner!—can
add serious spice to a restaurant meal. A sexy love note notifying
him of our exhausting plans for his member, dropped into our
man's briefcase, will surely give him something to think about as he
waits for the day to wind down.

But a guy with whom we have no firm lifetime commitment
best know that he needs to come with it, figure out new ways to
make our toes curl, make our throats hurt from screaming in pleasure, keep us guessing what he's going to do next to make us come
back for more—lest he get a wack grade in the bedroom department and, ultimately, a dropkick from the facilities.

See, we want some action. We've already established that there's only so much we can do to whip it on you; we think you all make it quite clear that it's okay for us to take the roller-coaster thrill ride with you, but that we can't exactly demonstrate that we know how to drive it without making you cock an eyebrow. So we recognize that, for a little while, we're going to have to simply ride shotgun.

And that's okay (for a little while, at least) if you know how to drive. If we are truly uninhibited, then we can trust that each sexual encounter will be an experience that we'll not only remember, but will keep us so incredibly excited that we won't be able to wait to get back over to your crib to create some more erotic memories.

It's important, though, that guys understand what constitutes creativity. It's not just your throwing my leg to a different direction every time we have sex, or your leading me to the kitchen today, the shower tomorrow, and the living-room sofa the next day. It's definitely not just your spreading chocolate on my breasts one day and then whipped cream two days later and then thinking your creative responsibilities are done.

Creativity for us means romantic.

Creativity for us means erotic.

Creativity for us means sensual.

Creativity means that the *entire night* is a new experience, not just the part that comes right before orgasm. That means that when we honor your invitation to your house, you surprise us with a beautiful candlelit dinner for two. That means that when you know we've had a hard day at work, you wow us with hot milk bubblebath to the sounds of Brian McKnight, then stand there at the ready with a towel to help us dry off when we're done soaking, and have enough muscles to carry us into the bedroom. That means that every once in a while, we'll get a summons at the job from our man telling us to meet you somewhere special, like that pretty hotel on the water or the parking lot of your old high school, or the swings in the playground near the pond in the next town over.

This is what will keep us coming back for more. Not to say that it takes the place of sex; we still need you to go to work in the boudoir—and we still want you to invite us to swing from the rafters. But we also need you to understand what is going to please us, what will have us running back to the girls and saying we got us a good one.

No, it's not something that you would have to do everytime we have sex; no one person is that damn energetic. But if you do it enough to create those memories and then turn us out sexually after that? Oh, you could probably, in the immortal words of the Artist Formerly Known as Prince, burn up your clothes, smash up your ride and I'd still come back for more.

It is, simply, the romance, followed by an evening of passionate lovemaking or mind-blowing sex. Trust me, you wouldn't be able to go wrong here.

Would you be insulted if we tried to give you some lessons in creativity?

From a Brother

Not if your suggestions were made with compassion and sensitivity. You must understand that we have grown up in a society that forces us to measure our manhood by the size of our members and the skill of our lovemaking. Just as it'd crush us if our lady laughed when she saw our organ for the first time, we'd also be devastated if she started barking out orders in the bedroom as if she can no longer stand our cluelessness.

As we discussed in the chapter on performance anxiety, we're terrified of being deemed unskilled in the bedroom. We have no accurate way of assessing our skill except for the feedback of our partners. We get most of our info about lovemaking techniques from superficial sources like books and movies, and we never really know whether we're doing it right unless somebody tells us. Many of us were lucky to have older experienced women early in our lives introduce us to the joy of pleasing and being pleased, kind of like sex tutorials. But there's always going to be a little sensitivity in this area.

When the suggestions are done the right way, they can be thrilling for us. We get to take a peek into our woman's libidinous thoughts, to see what kind of fuel gets her engine going. This is the kind of information that we crave but usually have a difficult time tracking down. A lot of our women evade questions about their sexual fantasies, I guess figuring that they could get into trouble if they offer their men such privileged glimpses at their fantasy life— we might get jealous or offended or even mad. All those possibilities do exist; our egos might not be able to take the information once we get it (like, did I really need to know that she liked Maxwell *that* much?), but we still covet it, even if it is risky for us.

How should the suggestions come? Well, if my lady tells me with a twinkle in her eye that it'd be a blast to go to Central Park and do it in a tree, I'm gonna be sprinting to find the car keys and my climbing shoes. If she says with a giddy smile that she bought some whipped cream while she was at the grocery store, I'm already going to be stripping down to transform myself into a sundae. If she tells me with a giggle that it feels wonderful when I suck her toes or lightly caress her nipples, I'm going to make sure I'm all over it the next time. It's much the same way we've always been told to discipline our children: Do it with positive reinforcement, not negative criticism. You pick out a time when the kiddies are doing something you like and you praise them effusively so they'll keep doing it. I hate to compare us to children, but I think there are some lessons there for grown folks to learn. In fact, we'd all be better off if that kind of positive reinforcement was used in most of our interactions with one another.

Masturbation

From a Sistah

My girlfriend Michelle found herself in a bit of trouble recently when she invited her man over and they got a little bit, well, let's just say "aggressive" in their lovemaking and the bed broke; her boyfriend offered to fix it and found her dildo between the mattresses.

> **Sex Tip:** Let us just say this: if you can watch each other masturbate, you deserve the Surgeon General Joycelyn Elders Award for Sexual Candor.

It wasn't pretty.

Needless to say, the bed didn't get fixed that night. Instead, boyfriend spent the next two hours grilling Michelle on her sexual proclivities and asking her what he was doing wrong that she felt it necessary to have sex without him.

"Ain't I good enough?" he asked, his eyes all wide and puppy-doggish, the rest of his face buried in his hands. "Why do you need that? You've got me."

It then quickly degenerated into questions on whether she'd been sleeping with someone else, if she'd ever had sex with other women, how many times she masturbated, when she masturbated, if she did it alone or with someone watching.

None of her answers, of course, was good enough. She might as well have been talking to the broken mattress.

Indeed, Michelle admitted that he was no slouch in the bed. Clearly, they at least had a healthy sexual relationship, one that was full of creativity and passion and pleasure. But her desire for creativity and passion and pleasure clearly extended well beyond the average three nights a week they found themselves busting up furniture. She was—is—sexual, likes how it feels, how it tastes, how it affects. And if she's in the mood to climb the walls and he's not around, she wasn't about to stop her groove on to wait for him to get over to her apartment.

He was shocked.

She didn't see why.

Isn't this, after all, what guys do? You all have bathrooms full of *Playboys*—um, and we know you're not reading them for just the "well-written articles," y'all—and shelves full of dirty videos. You seem to think about sex incessantly, and you ask for it—expect it—constantly. So we *know* if we're not in your bed, you're either with another woman (you better not be, though) or pleasuring yourself by yourself. We expect you to, really. May not like it in some cases, but expect it.

So why all the grief when *we* do it? Is it that shocking that we would want to keep ourselves, um, on our toes sexually, too? Do you all really think you've got the lock on what it takes to please women, and that no one else on this earth could possibly do it better than a man?

Well, let me break it down for ya, so that it will forever be broke: Women masturbate. They do it even though they have a man, and they do it especially when they don't have a man. Sometimes they're doing it because you're not getting the job done, sometimes they're doing it because, dammit, they just want to—no slight to you.

Simple as that.

Now, I don't know if homeboy was simply insecure when he practically accused Michelle of cheating on him by masturbating when he wasn't around, but we do get the sense that you all don't know very much about what we do to please ourselves sexually when we don't have a man. We kinda get the sense that you all think cobwebs are growing over our vaginas, and they don't get swept away until we invite a new, um, housecleaner into our lives.

Yeah.

Part of that is both our fault; we hardly talk about sex, except when we're having it, and so it's only natural that we wouldn't be privy to our partner's practices when you all are not in our bed. And let's not forget that we're only one step away from the time when we preached that masturbation was an abomination against God—or that it would at least make your hands hairy and your dick swell up and fall off.

Of course, when we grow up, we learn better. But sex talk is still liable to get us into a world of trouble, as we're sure homeboy doesn't really want to hear what we've all done and with whom we've done it—even if it was a one-person show.

So we kinda expect that you really don't want to hear that we masturbate on the regular, and enjoy it like a mug. Basically, we don't get the sense that you all think any different than Michelle's man.

Would you be upset if you found out I masturbate without you?

From a Brother
I don't think so. I think most men are extremely excited and pumped by the idea of their lady being so horny and sensual that she sometimes pleasures herself. We have always gotten the sense that masturbation was predominantly a male domain, that women frowned on it and thought perverse thoughts about us because we were such frequent practitioners. If we made the discovery that we were with a woman who had no such inhibitions about pleasuring herself, I think we'd figure that our own sexual encounters with her were bound to only get hotter and hotter.

Some of us—perhaps this was the case with your friend Michelle's man—might be a little worried if we saw that she was getting assistance in her self-pleasuring from some mammoth dildo, a loaded cannon that made our piece look like a pop gun. We might wonder how we'd fill her quota—if you know what I mean—if she's used to being packed to the gills. We might be a little anxious that she preferred her plastic paramour to our real-life flesh and bone. But those worries are usually far outweighed by our excitement over her enthusiatic cravings.

I can't even imagine the thrill we'd get from stumbling upon her in the act. It'd be one of the those intensely memorable erotic moments, the kind we'd be able to recall in vivid detail thirty years later—and we don't have a whole lot of those over the course of thirty years, either. Talk about memory enhancers—that one would be a memory detonator. We'd probably be embarrassed and a bit guilty and uncomfortable if we caught her, but we'd also practically be faint with excitement.

Of course, there's always a possibility that she's thinking about someone else as she masturbates, that she's doing a little fantasy partner self-pleasuring. If we had some way of proving that, it'd be immensely disturbing to us—we might not ever recover. But the beauty of prancing around in a fantasy world is that it's all ours, off-limits to anyone and everyone else, including our significant other. And it should stay that way—even if we stress you for weeks to find out what you think about when you masturbate, if your answer is apt to be anything other than "Why, I think about you, of course, dahling" you should tell us to mind our own damn business. Actually, on second thought, don't even tell us that—it's bound to arouse suspicion. Tell us you were thinking about our next get-together. It will inspire us to new heights. You won't be sorry.

The problem most of us, male and female, have with masturbation is that we are so thoroughly indoctrinated by the idea that it is dirty and reprehensible that we have a difficult time getting past our shame and guilt. Every time we think about it, along with the tingles comes a twinge of embarrassment. We are being bad boys or bad girls. People will think something is wrong with us if they find out. A part of us may even believe just a tiny bit that something *is* wrong with us. With much of our sexuality we harbor that creeping fear that we are abnormal—this is probably exacerbated with masturbation because it is one of the few sexual acts that has been described as wrong to us from the time we were knee-high to a grasshopper. With boys, our shame about it was always so profound that we'd come up with dozens of derogatory names for it to protect ourselves, as if we were somehow insulated from the possibility of ridicule if God and everybody else heard how derisively we referred to masturbation. Choking the chicken, spanking the monkey, beating your meat, beating off, whacking off . . . the names go on and on. And they're all boy names describing boy acts. Growing up, I never heard a name for girl masturbation. I don't even think I was aware of the possibility that girls masturbated. It was nowhere near my radar screen. So as an adult, finding out my woman pleasured herself would be like walking into a room and catching my woman screaming at the Jets quarterback for taking the sack instead of throwing out of bounds, or yelling at the Yankees shortstop for looking at a 3–2 fastball down the middle. It would be a shock that brought me unlimited joy to find out we had this big gigantic thing in common.

How would you feel if you found out your man masturbates without you?

From a Sistah

It would be easy for me to sit here and say, "Honey, it's okay—go on ahead and slang yo' thang. After all, it's yours." But nah—there's a much bigger part of me that's bothered by the thought of my man pleasuring himself without me.

Childish and insecure as it is, I feel the same way that Michelle's man does: If you're pulling your own chain, then I must not be getting the job done—because if I was, you wouldn't find it necessary to do yourself. My creativity, my liveliness, my excitability, my straight-up skills would be more than sufficient, making it so that you really don't have the time, desire, or inclination to have sex with anybody—including yourself—but me.

I wouldn't say it's tantamount to cheating or anything like that; that would be a bit much, even for me. But there is a certain level of imagination that goes into masturbation—and there is certainly, in some cases, a need for tools, like X-rated magazines, videos, or pictures, in order for a person to reach that climax. That means that you could possibly be thinking about a sexual escapade that doesn't involve me, that involves, say, a vivid replay of the time you and your ex-girlfriend (that would be the one whose picture I, um, stumbled across in your keepsake box) had sex on the empty Brooklyn-bound subway car à la *Risky Business,* and she made you holler so loud they heard you all the way up in the Bronx. It means that you could very well be looking at the naked hootchies spreading their legs for the cameras of *Players* magazine. You could be thinking about the stripper who has a couple of your hard-earned dollars stuffed down her panties, or one of those women in the porn movie you keep tucked away at the back of your closet.

Bottom line is, you could be thinking about someone other than me.

I don't like that.

I want to be your fantasy. The moment you're so horny a girl could think you have a roll of quarters stuffed down your crotch, I want to be the one you run to. I want to be the one to tease you, please you, and leave you with nothing but satisfaction. I want to be the one who feels needed.

Besides, doesn't masturbation whittle down the intimate

moments that we would normally share together? Say, for instance, you masturbated, like, three times a week. Doesn't that lead to your deciding, for at least three days out of that week that, because you've made yourself come, you don't have to have sex with me? Doesn't that mean that I'm losing out on a good time, too? Or that I'm left to pleasure myself because I'm not getting enough satisfaction my damn self?

Your masturbating means you've searched for and found that satisfaction somewhere else, and now you're going to come to me all empty-handed, uninspired, drained, and used-up. It makes me feel, well, irrelevant.

This, of course, doesn't apply in all cases. In fact, there are a few instances where I would fully accept your masturbating. As I write this, I'm nine months pregnant—have a baby in my belly the size of several basketballs. I waddle. My thighs rub together. My breasts leak. And no matter how many times my husband tells me I'm just as sexy pregnant as not, I still have my days—shoot, let me stop sugarcoating it; I've had months—when sex is the furthest thing from my mind. I ain't thinking about spreading my legs, I ain't thinking about oral sex, I ain't thinking about hand jobs. I'm thinking about fetal movements, baby room decorations, and sleep—lots of it. And our sex life has suffered for it, as Nick and I are two very sexual people who—I like to think at least—had a pretty slamming sex life before the lil' miss made her presence increasingly known.

If Nick's masturbating, I certainly understand.

I would also understand if my back was out of whack and I was out of commission for a while, or if I was on my deathbed.

But that's it.

The rest of the time, I want to be the one to handle that, baby.

And if you're in the mood and I'm not, tomorrow is certainly another day.

Do guys continue to masturbate as much as they did when they didn't have a steady partner?

From a Brother

No, we don't. Even if we wanted to, the logistics of a relationship would likely allow less time and opportunity to spend some quality intimate time with ourselves. But for most us, the truth is that we don't want to as much anymore. As long as we feel our sexual needs are being met—or almost met—we don't need to as much anymore.

Throughout the years, we have developed quite a complicated, multilayered relationship with masturbation. We've been captivated by our organ since before we even went to school, knowing that just a gentle touch felt strangely pleasurable. After our first wet dream, that captivation soon bordered on obsession: we couldn't get enough of the explosive joy we had the power to make ourselves feel. It was almost like discovering a free and potent new drug that we had unfettered access to in unlimited supply. We became just as fascinated by the gifts that our own organ offered as by the undiscovered mysteries of the female organ. Yeah, we soon found out our member can be overly temperamental and sometimes even too picky, but that didn't diminish our love for him and our conviction to do anything—almost including give our life—to protect him.

Masturbation has always been a reliable friend, a comforting presence in those lean high school and college years, later becoming an old buddy whom we're still very fond of but we just don't need to visit with as much anymore. But we never desert the buddy completely. He will always have a purpose in our life. Sometimes he has many purposes.

When we first start to become sexually active, masturbation can be a valuable tool as a **premature ejaculation suppressor**. If we think we might wind up in bed with a new woman and we're so nervous about the encounter and so horny that we suspect we might blast off way too early, a visit with our old friend just before the date begins will calm us down and improve our chances later on of lasting until the deed is done and delighting our new woman with our stamina and staying power. Of course, once we become accustomed to her and we're not so horny and excited anymore, we no longer need the premature ejaculation suppressor.

But now we might need the old friend for **impulse control**. If the boss's secretary oozes sexuality from every pore and insists on wearing skintight sweater dresses every day, no bra, and panties tiny enough to give a clear view of the wedgie riding up her ass, then we might need some impulse control. Even though we have a partner now, the situation may call for us to rush into a bathroom stall and revisit our old buddy once in a while so that we can remain impervious to her many charms. So that we can protect our relationship at home. So that we don't mess up. Impulse control is important.

As is the **stress reliever**. The job has been beating our ass regularly, we come home drowning in anxiety every night, we need to take matters into our hands. Most of us don't have a masseuse on staff at home to attack that stress, but we do have our left (or right) hand. And it's cheaper.

Janet Jackson is probably never going to knock on our apartment door wearing those tight jeans and that dark halter top she paraded around in with Djimon Honsou and that white boy in the "Love Will Never Do" video. We'd probably win the lottery two weeks in a row before that happened. But with the use of our old buddy, we can have wild, passionate encounters with our whole starting lineup of fantasy partners. It may or may not please Janet or Vanessa Williams or Jennifer Lopez or Lisa Nicole Carson—am I revealing a little too much here about my fantasy life?—to know that they are regularly putting in starring performances all over the country with no compensation, but now they know why we pay such close attention to the videos and movies they *do* get paid for. We're doing research to help out an old friend.

While hearing about the fantasy partner may not thrill our real-life partners, they might like to know that masturbation can also serve as our **memory enhancer**. This use is activated when we've just had the most fantastic lovemaking session with our lady, we return home to our apartment, and the whole incredible evening is replayed in our minds as we stretch out on our beds. We picture our lady's dangerous curves, the way she moved, the way she felt, and we use our old friend to enhance the replaying in our mind and help us revisit some of the sensations we were having at the time. We probably do this less and less over the years, but it can still occur even if our lady sleeps inches away from us and we have been married for many years.

Although we are so intimately familiar with the little friend between our legs that we know exactly how he likes to be treated, our own hand can't hold a candle to the excitement we feel when our lady decides to do the deed for us. In a way, that can feel almost more intimate than intercourse itself because she is subjugating her own pleasure to focus on ours. When she's done, we feel so eternally grateful that we might insist on returning the favor.

CHAPTER 18

Porn, Strip Clubs, and All Manner of Freakiness

From a Sistah

They don't talk about it much—at least not with us. It's like a secret world that we aren't privy to, a seedy underworld of big booties and leather and stilettos and weaves and fake double-Ds and cheap perfume and dollar-store makeup. And like every woman inhabiting it is a nasty freak mama willing to shake her fat ass in my man's face for his amusement and sexual satisfaction—and, of course, his hard-earned dollar (literally).

And we're not supposed to be bothered by any of it.

We're also, I guess, not supposed to be bothered when, in the

Sex Tip: Okay, if you keep having Vanessa Williams–Jayne Kennedy–Pamela Anderson flashbacks and you just can't bring yourself to star in your own homemade porn flick, you and your partner can still leap into the sex industry together. You can do stripteases for each other. And not just a few wiggles while you tear off the dress and sit on his face: we're talking the stripper music, the stripper/ Chippendales outfit, and at least enough stripper moves to get a few dollar bills tucked into your drawers.

middle of the evening, while we're minding our business like we usually do, we get a phone call from some chick named Heather, talking about how she needs to leave a message for our mates—"Could you just tell him," she asks in that stupid, girly, Betty Boop voice, "that his *Playboy* subscription is about to run out and we have a special offer for him to renew it?"—and, um, we never knew boyfriend was reading the damn thing, let alone getting it delivered to the house.

And Lord forbid we object to Valentine's gifts of freak gear, matchbooks advertising Steam Heat and The Players' Club, and XXX movies in the brown paper video store bag, when we told you at least five times before you left that we wanted you to pick up *love jones.*

Now, admittedly, there are plenty of women out there who aren't bothered by it at all. In fact, some of them may be downright turned on by it—go arm-in-arm with their men to the strip club, read all the "great articles" in *Playboy,* and fix the popcorn and get the beer while the VCR is cueing up *Buffy Does the Football Squad.*

But you know what? Some of us do get bothered by it—can't stand it, even. Can't take driving past the parking lot of the local strip club, listening to the moans of the women in the porn tape, thinking about the men who are turned on by nipple rings and leather whips. It is embarrassing for some women to watch other people do all kinds of things with their body that, had they been in Sodom and Gomorrah, would have earned them a warm spot in the fire. For some other women, it's taken as a sign of their own inadequacies when it comes to their performance in the sack, like the only reason he's watching this is because she's not handling her business in the bedroom. Still others think it's simply a sin.

But that doesn't seem to bother as many men as it does women. Y'all get turned on just thinking about it, sneaking out with the boys to see it, talking about it with one another in hushed tones and code words, thinking we don't get what you're grinning about. I had a girlfriend who ended up kicking her man to the curb because boyfriend was spending more time in the booty bars, giving away all his little money, than he was at her house. He'd be there basically every Thursday and Saturday night with the boys, coming home drunk, smelling like smoke, clothes all sweated-out and stuff, like he was putting in some hard work or something. She figured that any man who spent more money on and time with some stage heifer than he did with her should go on ahead and live and sleep with the heifer rather than up in her house. He argued that it was all just innocent fun—that he and the boys were just out having a good time. "It's not like I'm cheating on you or anything," he told her over and over again. "It's just entertainment."

Well, we can think of a billion other ways men can entertain themselves that don't involve naked women, sex, and all manners of freakiness. Let's see—there's the movies, there's bowling, there's tennis, there's long walks in the park, there's Scrabble, there's reading, there's TV, there's the mall. Well, maybe not the mall. But you get the drift.

I take it, though, that the kind of entertainment you're looking for doesn't quite fit into that "family" kind of fun, the kind that you can let your mama participate in if she happened to be in town. And we just do not get why. So, could you help us out? **Why is it necessary to partake in that kind of entertainment? Should I take it as an insult if you're at the booty club every weekend?**

From a Brother

At its core, all this stuff is merely erotica: instruments to enhance or initiate sexual pleasure. No person can really decide what forms of erotica are necessary or superfluous for someone else—it's all so personal and subjective. One man's kinky is another man's corny. But I believe there is a line separating acceptable erotica from unacceptable obsession, the kind that you should find insulting. Usually we are able to find that line ourselves, but some of us may need someone else—such as a spouse—to do it for us.

In indulging our erotic tastes, we must answer a key question: How much sociability do we seek? Do we want to involve our partner in viewing the porno tapes? Would we prefer to go to the booty bar with our boys rather than by ourselves? Does our partner share our interest in leather, or at least does she know about it? Have we told her about our butt plug? Does she know how much we like pain?

If we can answer yes to the question of sociability, it means we haven't allowed our interest to become obsession; our erotic life hasn't gotten so seedy and debased that we're ashamed to let anybody know about it. That's important, because it's less likely to be a danger to our union if it's something that our partner knows about and at least tacitly approves of. It's when the stuff becomes so secret and so shameful that we have to sneak around to indulge in it that we get into trouble.

For instance, if a guy's most overwhelming fantasy has always been to have two women at the same time or to make love to a total stranger, he's only inviting trouble if he goes out there and tries to bring it to life behind his partner's back. But if he finds a way to tell her (he gets major props just for finding the nerve), he might get the shock of his life as she responds that she's always wanted the same thing, or she might say she'd be willing to help him act it out. The point is, once we go public with these thoughts they are less likely to grow into obsessions and less likely to lead to calamity.

Our sexuality is a complex creature, fed by isolated events from our past, formed by various and sundry characters who have walked (or crept) in and out of our lives, nurtured by sometimes strange and inexplicable mental connections between our inner erotic world and the humdrum outer world, inflamed by the individuality of personal taste and preference. Not only is it distasteful, but also illogical to impose any moral code we might have fashioned over the years on another person's sexuality, as long as that person isn't breaking any laws or hurting anyone. This applies to everything from homosexuality to a predilection for sniffing dirty panties. Therefore, to ask another person why any particular part of his or her sexual makeup is necessary is no different from asking why he walks the way he does or she laughs the way she does. We have as much control over the things we find erotic or stimulating as we do over the smells we like or the foods we crave.

As for the second part of your question, if I'm at the booty bar every weekend, you've told me to stop and I ignore you, then yes, you should definitely be insulted. Under that scenario, I have a problem that needs to be addressed. Either the problem is with you or there's a sensual, nubile, and incredibly flexible young creature down at the booty bar from whom I just can't pry myself away. In either case, we need to talk immediately to figure out what's happening. I'm not trying to suggest that this is going to be an easy conversation—if I'm trying to get away from you, I'm probably not going to be eager to tell you; if I've become obsessed with some big booty stripper, I'm probably going to be even less eager to tell you. When these erotic interests get to the point where they are interfering with our relationship, they become more than mere sexual propensities, they become distractions, obstacles.

On the other hand, if I go to the booty bar every once in a while with some friends, you shouldn't feel insulted. These occasions aren't much different than us going out drinking and looking at all the pretty girls. The presence of other guys acts as a buffer, a deterrent to any real trouble coming to find us. We're not likely to go anywhere with anybody or do anything more than a harmless table dance if our boys are around. I think many women over the years have developed a misplaced mistrust in these boys' nights out, thinking we're going to be engaged in all sorts of hedonistic pursuits. In actuality, I think guys are more likely to protect one another from going too far or doing something we'll later regret. If they know we're deeply in love with the woman of our dreams, they're going to stop us from messing all that up in a wild, drunken stupor. Our boys are not the enemy—more than likely, they got your back.

Why are women more judgmental or inhibited about exploring the outer limits of sexual satisfaction and arousal?

From a Sistah
Inhibited? I don't think so.

Just because we don't want to watch Janet Jackme take it up the butt—I never thought I'd do this, but to quote the legendary nasty girl Lil' Kim, "yeah, yeah what"—doesn't mean we don't want to, aren't capable of, and never will be sexually excitable or interesting. We love making love, we love pleasing our men, we love making sure that we are pleased in return—and creativity is just as important to us as it is to you. Those who are inhibited are strictly missionary, once every other week, specifically for procreation purposes. Prudes, most of us are not.

But I'll certainly admit to our being judgmental. Don't we have the right to be? Most of the porn, most of the strip clubs, and most of the freakiness associated with the two of them center on what the man likes, not necessarily what we women would be interested in. That means that the Buttman series of porn movies centers on the way *her* ass looks while the two of them are having sex, the way *her* mouth looks when she's giving him oral sex, the way *her* breasts bounce while he's banging her from every which way. We're used to our body parts being put on display on the television shows and the magazines and the movies—tell me the last time, save for *NYPD Blue,* you've seen a man's butt or penis up in the camera or in a sexy mainstream picture—but we didn't quite expect that the porn movies would give unequal attention to our needs to see the booty, too. And don't get me started on the gratuitous women-on-women scenes. While they may turn you on, it's going to excite me about as much as two men screwing each other in front of the camera would excite you.

Get my point?

A lot of us also feel like the women who participate in these kinds of sexual activities are just some seedy, shady bitches who are either being taken advantage of and too stupid to realize it, or are simply on some mind-altering shit—maybe even without them knowing it or against their will—when they agree to shake their titties in front of a roomful of grown men. You know the horror stories: a fourteen-year-old girl runs away, gets turned out by the local Freddie Mac Pimp Trick Gangsta Clique, and, to make some money on the side—enough for some Cheerios and a cheap lace bra—she turns to taking her clothes off in front of a bunch of nasty, grubby, hairy men. I'm not saying that there aren't women who enjoy this profession and prosper in it; I'm sure there are plenty of women who have made a ton of money showing off their beautiful bodies and enjoying sex and becoming famous in the porn industry. But how many of them are actually happy with what they're doing—or aware of it, even? How many of them got caught up into something that they didn't bargain for, and are now being taken advantage of by a bunch of men—or women—profiting from something that is so precious to the rest of us and should be precious to them—sex? Would you want it to be your daughter or mother or sister in that movie or up on that stage?

I think not.

Quite frankly, one of the biggest reasons I'm against it is because I just don't get it. I mean, what's the fascination, anyway? It's a bunch of women dancing naked. You seen one, you've seen 'em all, as far as I'm concerned. For instance, I was assigned by the *Daily News* to cover an erotica expo at New York City's Jacob Javits Center once, and I have to admit, I was looking forward to seeing what the big deal was. Conservative groups were mad because it was being advertised on television and in the local newspapers and magazines, and a church group even canceled its own convention because it didn't want to be in the same building as an expo full of whips, chains, and XXX videos. I figured they were going to show me something I needed to see, something that would turn me on, something I could bring home to Papa.

No dice.

What I got was a bunch of pictures of women in various stages of undress, breasts hanging out of latex and leather, whips between their lips, red pumps hiked up on chairs. Did nothing for me. I saw chocolate penises, vaginas, and breasts that cost upward of fifteen dollars. Did nothing for me. I saw vendors selling erotic books. I have some of them; don't need any more. I saw other vendors selling overpriced black rubber clothing—one was selling rubber thongs for fifty dollars—neck collars with spikes, whips, and other various torture devices, and a bunch of dirty movies. Whoop-dee-doo. I just couldn't control my excitement.

I'm being facetious.

I have no interest in whips and chains and latex thongs and pictures of big-breasted blond women. It just doesn't turn me on. So why would I all of a sudden get excited because you brought one home?

In fact, if you brought a XXX tape home, or you were looking in *Playboy* every time I saw you going into the bathroom, I'd be more inclined to take it as an insult. Why? Because I would assume that you're not happy with what I'm doing for you—that what we do together is somehow inadequate. If I'm taking care of business, you don't need to look at naked women in a magazine, or get yourself excited over another woman getting sexed before you get horny for me—at least that's how we women feel. If you have to depend on other women to get your erection, then you come lie down next to me, the first thing I'm going to assume is that you're not thinking about me—you're thinking about her. That doesn't make us feel good. In fact, it makes us feel like shit.

I don't think this would prove a useful tool to liven up our sex lives; in fact, I think it would pose serious problems for it, as I would constantly feel that inadequacy creeping up—would constantly wonder if you're thinking about her rather than me. It would always get in the way of my enjoyment—and if only one of us is getting something out of it, well, Houston? Problem.

We'd figured you'd know this by now. We certainly expect that you would understand when we do not want to participate in it, and why we don't necessarily want you to, either. But some men continue to do so, even when they know we don't like it. And we don't quite understand that one.

If I'm not with it and you know it makes me upset, would you stop it to save the relationship? Or, if I ask you to, would that be a deal breaker?

From a Brother

If it bothers you and you ask us to stop, most likely we will. We might not be real happy about it, but we'd have to be pretty far gone with our obsession to pick it over our relationship.

Of course, what we prefer is that you understand where we're coming from and you allow us to indulge our preferences, as long as we do it within moderation. But sometimes that's not possible. Some women consider any form of pornography to be sexist and exploitative of women, no matter how many times the "actresses" on the tapes come forward to say they willingly chose their line of work, so there's not much in this area they'd be willing to tolerate. And they certainly wouldn't be down with watching the movies with their man. If they're especially condemning and judgmental, they'll consider us a partner in the exploitation by our viewing of a movie. Feminist literature is crammed with studies and statements reporting that using pornography makes men more callous, distrustful, and violent toward women—even makes men more likely to rape. So everything and anything that would get a triple-X slapped on it becomes pornography, with no effort made to categorize, to label, to differentiate. Ironically, the stock-in-trade of all soap operas and any romantic movie geared toward women is the steamy love scene, when the woman is swept into the man's arms and they engage in a passionate kiss that leads to passionate sex while the soulful saxophone plays in the background. Apparently these are all okay—but let the camera slide down and show a penis and a vagina . . . and suddenly any men who happen to be viewing will be transformed into boorish, callous rapists. Sure, some porn is sick and degrading, but must everything that is explicit be lumped together, making any young girl who grows up repeatedly hearing such arguments scared to death of all porn and any men inclined to watch it? Whether you realize it or not, not all pornography is the same. There are even movies out there produced by women with the intent of being viewed by couples. Imagine that. Candida Royale and her Femme Productions have become quite well known, producing scores of movies with the female libido in mind—the romantic plotlines, longer-building climaxes, and camera angles that give equal time to showing the woman's pleasure are all designed to appeal to women as well as men.

Would such a hard-line stance from our women ever be a deal breaker? Speaking for myself, if it became clear to me that her inflexibility in this area was illustrative of an unbending personality in many other areas, I'd start to get worried. There aren't many traits that will lead to the collapse of a relationship faster than inflexibility. I mean, how presumptuous is it for us to expect that our partner is going to see every issue the way we do and, if they don't, be willing abruptly to change their views to agree with ours? Just because she thinks that a particular form of sexual expression is wrong or not acceptable doesn't mean we're going to be coming from the same place. You'd think most women would understand and abide by that. But I'm sure many don't—and, as a result, many men are out there hiding their sexual fantasies or erotic interests and feeling bad and dirty about it.

If her desire to keep me away from the erotic activity wasn't part of an overall pattern, then I'd probably go along with her wishes, as long as I felt they were within reason. That last part of the sentence is important. If oral sex is important to me and I start moving my mouth down to her southern regions during lovemaking, I might start having second thoughts about the future of the relationship if I'm greeted with a loud "Eeeww! That's disgusting!"

What to Do When You Don't Wanna

From a Sistah

It was, perhaps, *the* single most grueling day you'd ever had.

It started with the pantyhose—the run just kept getting bigger and longer and nastier-looking as you ran, in your heels, to catch the train to work. You missed it. You waited a half hour for the next one, and not a single solitary one of the men on the train offered you a seat, so you stood with the rest of the women, holding and grabbing onto anything to keep from falling as the conductor took the curves like a madman. You walked the fifteen blocks to work, in the rain, because the same men who wouldn't give

Sex Tip: If he/she says no but your loins say go, your options are few. Try this one on: Close the bathroom door, drop your drawers, and handle your business yo' damn self (see Chapter 17). Remember: Before you had each other, you had you. If you still need contact with your partner, crawl into bed, wrap your arms around him/her, and tell him/her why you love him/her so much. You may be pleasantly surprised by how your affection inspires him/her.

you a seat on the train beat you to the taxi line, and you couldn't hitch a ride if you were Pamela Anderson pre–bust reduction.

Of course, because you walked, you were late for the big meeting you'd scheduled with the client you thought was going to get you the deal that would make you look like superwoman. Didn't go over too well. Forget the raise, the promotion, and the congratulatory party; get to work because the boss is going to be in your booty for the next week, imploring you to seal the deal *or else.*

You get home three hours after you'd usually get there and arrive to a mailbox full of bills, an answering machine full of messages from girlfriends who all think their problems need handling *now,* and a refrigerator with nothing in it but leftover sesame beef from last week's Chinese restaurant excursion.

It's been just that kinda day.

And now, your mate is knocking on the door with a hard-on that would rival that of Marky Mark's prosthetic in *Boogie Nights.*

You know what he wants: sex.

You know what you want: sleep. Lots of it.

But your recounting of the day from hell you had, the broke-down look you've assumed, the constant yawns escaping your lips—none of that really registers with him, and he keeps trying to head toward the bedroom. The concept "not tonight, honey" isn't registering, despite the obvious signs.

What's wrong with y'all?

This plays itself out in all kinds of ways, on all kinds of days; we make it obvious we don't want to; you keep pushing. Like, how many of us can identify with the middle-of-the-night rub, the one where you're just getting good into your sleep, drooling and carrying on, hugged-up on the pillow and just straight-up *out,* and all of a sudden, out of nowhere, like a nightmare, you feel hot air on your ears, probing fingers, and other body parts on your back, your breasts, your butt.

Try to say, "Baby—I'm sleep." It's dark as hell—pitch-black—in the room, but you can still make out the puppy-dog eyes and the three-year-old pout mouth he's giving you when you make it clear you're not interested in nookie right now.

You might as well have told him that you're not interested in nookie *ever.*

We simply don't understand this thing, this attitude when we don't feel like putting out. I mean, tomorrow is another day, right? People get tired, people don't feel well, people just don't *feel* like it sometimes. My husband may not want to admit this, but he's good for making you feel, like, guilty for not being in the mood when he's in the mood. Like, when I was pregnant, the last thing on my mind was bonin', okay? I mean, like, for the first four months, morning sickness had me going one-on-one with the porcelain god all day long, then for the next few months—which came during the winter—I was sick with the flu and colds for almost the entire season, and then for the last few months, I just didn't feel like it. It hurt. It was uncomfortable. My belly was in the way.

Sex was rare.

And I felt bad about it, no lie. Because my husband is an extremely sexual human being—as am I. Before the pregnancy, we had an awesome sex life—but hey, certain things change other things, and in our case, pregnancy certainly turned our sex lives upside down. Boyfriend would mope around the house, kiss me, then, five minutes later, tell me "You know, if we weren't pregnant, we would have been having sex right now." On another occassion, he pulled a muscle in his butt while playing tennis, and his best friend implored him to get me to massage it, to make the boo-boo better. My husband informed me that they immediately started joking that he shouldn't tease himself like that, as he knew that the moment he got excited, he'd be excited by his damn self.

Lord, did I feel bad—but I would have felt worse if I had sex with him just to please him. I mean, shouldn't everybody be satisfied?

That doesn't appear to cross brothers' minds, though. It's like we have purposely denied you nookie to make you feel bad. Perhaps you can explain this to us: **Why do you guys take it personal when we say we're not interested in sex tonight? What's up with the attitude?**

From a Brother

Attitude? *What* attitude? *Are you talking about the way we react when you turn your back on the man you love, giving him a close-up of your ratty head rag, when he's primed and poised to pour his entire being into the one thing for which he has dedicated his life—making you happy—while hitting so many of your special places that you get cramps in your esophagus from screaming so loud? Is that the attitude to which you refer? Oh.*

As I've said before, just because we're married doesn't mean we can't get our feelings hurt from rejection. In fact, we're probably even *more* likely to get our feelings hurt. I know this may be hard for you, but try putting yourselves in our position for just a minute: We get home from a day of stress and hard labor just aching to lay our eyes on the woman we love. You have arrived there before us and already made yourself comfortable by removing everything except perhaps your bra and panties. They may even be those lacy, sheer, and sexy-as-hell panties and bra. The ones you know for a fact make us think nasty thoughts. You might be standing in front of the stove (or microwave) or maybe just sitting on the couch flipping through the channels. You look about as tasty as a peach cobbler, and just as rich and juicy. Right away we've caught an express train to Boner City. And we stay there in Boner for the rest of the night, practically drooling on ourselves every time you pass by our line of sight. You may even be oblivious to the effect you're having on us, though I suspect not. At this moment, the passionate muscle memory of every one of our hundreds or thousands of sexual encounters is surging through us, almost making us weak. We become focused on one thing only: to get the booty.

We may have been thinking about it all day, remembering how beautiful it looked propped up and wiggling in front of our face the last time we did it. How soft and round it was. How much we loved the way the breasts jutted out as you fed them to us. Damn, how could we forget an image like that? All the sexual encounters in the future, all the tomorrows, are of no consequence to us because we crave it *now*. At some point you take off the bra and slide a T-shirt over your torso, but we can see the butt cheeks peeking out from below the hem—and, of course, as is your usual custom, you're sporting a massive wedgie—and we can watch the nipples poking through. Surely you can sense our hunger, the fever in our eyes, the shortness of our breath when you bend over to pick up the fallen napkin. You are a walking and talking Venus, a seductive and celestial body oozing sensuality from every pore, cramming it all up in our face. Hours pass, meals are eaten, if there are kids involved they've been put down for the night, and we make our way to the bedroom. We are tingling. We know it's gonna be so damn good. We slip into the bathroom to brush our teeth—we want the breath to be extra sweet-smelling. We step back into the room, so eager and ready . . . and you're about two seconds from slumber. We snuggle up next to you, press our boner into your butt, maybe thrust it forward a few times. Nothing. You moan something about being beat, about needing sleep. As if the twenty or thirty minutes our lovemaking would take would render you useless the next day. As if it's not important to you that I've spent the last twelve hours dreaming about this moment. As if any of us are guaranteed tomorrow. Now do you understand?

If you say you don't wanna, should we try to get you in the mood or just give up?

From a Sistah

Two things that annoy the mess out of me: the sound of a mosquito buzzing around my ear while I'm trying to sleep, and the feel of a hard-on pressed into my back while I'm trying to sleep.

At least I can kill the mosquito.

This is something we women just don't get—guys' inability to take no for an answer. It's like, which part of the letters N and O didn't you understand?

Let us make it crystal for ya: When we say we don't want to, we don't want to. No, you should not assume that we really mean yes, and we're just making it a little more interesting for you by playing hard to get. No, you should not assume that a little poking and prodding will be the perfect elixir to get us out of funk mode and into the mood. No, the puppy-dog eyes *do not* work; they simply make us want to roll up the newspaper and swat you with it. Hard.

It's not easy saying no to you guys; you all are so good at making women—particularly your mates—feel guilty if you aren't bonin' on the regular, and the last thing we want you to think is that we're selfish, nonsexual prudes. We know how important sex is to you, and we certainly don't need you searching for it elsewhere.

But it's important that you understand that we like it, too—just not all the time. Just because you've been sitting around for the past twelve hours thinking about all the things you want to do to us in the sack doesn't mean that we were, too. To assume that would be just as silly as your thinking that just because you were in the mood for Japanese, I should want some sushi, too. Simply put, people have different tastes and feelings and moods—and no matter how much they know about each other or how long they've been together, they're not always going to be on the same page.

Particularly when it comes to sex.

We're not saying no just for the sake of saying no or to hurt your feelings. (Of course, there are some instances where sex is used as a bargaining tool—denied if you don't act right, given if you do—but only the fast-assed high school girls practice that one on the regular. Well, them and extremely immature women who stupidly do not recognize that they will be spotted out quick, fast, and in a hurry by the more alert brothers.) We are saying no because we just don't feel like it. It's not a difficult concept to grasp if you're a woman: I don't feel like washing my hair today, because I'm not in the mood for all the tugging and pulling and sitting; I don't feel like going grocery shopping today, because I'm not in the mood for all the searching and the standing and the waiting in line; I don't feel like having sex today, because I'm not in the mood for the kissing and the hugging and the thrusting and the pounding. I just want to go to sleep. Damn.

That's not to say we're equating sex with chores; for most of us, there is no better pleasure than being with a man who makes our toes curl.

But there are days when we'd rather just go on ahead and get our toes massaged, then roll over and go to sleep. And if we tell you this, we expect you to respect that—to understand that N-O means, simply, no. Your trying to push past that is a bore; your succeeding in pushing past our no turns the sex into a chore, because it then becomes us simply spreading our legs to shut you up and make you happy, not necessarily ourselves.

And I know that you know (because you've said this to me before) that there's nothing more unsatisfying than sex with a woman who simply lies there and lets you use her as a receptacle for your bodily fluids.

Now there are instances when, if you tried a little harder, you could get some. Those instances, however, do not come after she has actually said no. They come when you're hugging her and she hugs you back, then you kiss her and she kisses you back, then you rub her and she rubs you back, then you finger her and she fingers you back—you get the picture. You may have had to make the first moves, but she's following along with you—lock and step—making it plainly obvious that she's with it if you are.

But, again, if you hug her and she hugs you back, and you kiss her and she kisses you back, then you rub her and she says, "You know what, baby? I'm not in the mood," then you need to back up, zip up, shut up, and get over it.

After all, there's always tomorrow.

What's the best way to tell you without hurting your feelings that I just don't want to tonight?

From a Brother

You could give me something to look forward to. We could make a date for the next day, perhaps in the middle of the afternoon if it's a weekend, or on our lunch break, or as soon as we get home, or as soon as the kids are in bed, when we will get together and explore the bounds of our passion. There is nothing quite like anticipation, which is what I tried to demonstrate with my previous answer. A marriage is about familiarity and comfort, but it's also about anticipation. We need to always have something that we're looking forward to, some excitement that gets the spine to tingling.

If you really want to make things easy on me, you could borrow a page from the Vatican's College of Cardinals. You could utilize the fireplace and send smoke up through the chimney on nights when I'm going to get some; no smoke on nights when nothing's happening. That way as I'm driving up to the house I'll know whether I should put my anticipation on hold. I'm sure I'll still visit Boner City, but I'll know I won't be sampling the local fare while I'm there. It would also be especially considerate on your part if you wore flannel neck-to-toe pajamas around the house on those nights when there was no smoke. And put the ratty head rag on right after you get home. And take out the contact lenses right away and put on the old glasses, the cheap ones with the extra-thick lenses and the black frames. While you're at it, you might want to eat a lot of onions and garlic for dinner—and don't worry about the unpleasant taste in your mouth afterward; I'm sure your breath will smell fine.

If we don't have a fireplace, perhaps we could invest in a flag-pole for the front lawn. That way, you could run a red flag up there on the nights when you wanna bone and a white flag when the proceedings will be as bland as vanilla. Or we could buy one of those neon lights that they have outside of diners. We wouldn't need anything fancy—just the OPEN and CLOSED signs. I think they'd be self-explanatory.

Teenagers

From a Sistah

It was just the way it was going to be.

Daddy said I couldn't date until I was married, and I wasn't allowed to get married until I was well into my forties. Who was I to question him? Both my father and best friend, Jimmy Millner, was one of the two people on this earth—his wife, my mother, Bettye would be the other—whom I'd consistently listened to and obeyed during my short years on this earth. His order didn't make much sense if I thought about it hard enough; how in the hell was I supposed to get hitched if I couldn't go through the natural progression toward matrimony, the chief step being dating a person of the opposite sex?

I looked at my father like he had two sets of eyes and a horn growing out of his forehead, laughed like a maniac, and happily trotted off to the kitchen to get a snack and finish up my homework. I mean, it wasn't like I, already in eleventh grade and still dateless, much less boyfriendless, was getting any play anyway. Sure, I had people I admired, but I'd never come close to having a boyfriend. Well, maybe once.

His name was Shawn, and he was cute, I guess—tall, dark, with these really pretty thick, bushy eyebrows. And he was nice, too—the first guy who ever paid me any kind of mind. Used to stick around after school, before his basketball practice, to talk to him and giggle and (kinda) gaze into his eyes. I thought it would turn into something, like maybe my first kiss, but my alleged-turned-former best friend got to him (just like she did with every other guy I'd remotely shown an interest in at Brentwood High School) first. Kissed him, made it real clear she was willing to give it up, and got his nose wide open before I could say the first word in. "But damn—can't I get some?"

I was pitiful like that; wrapped up into the books, afraid of boys, and scared to death of the prospect of getting pregnant and becoming, like, a complete and total high school loser. The extent of my dating came in fantasies. They consisted of my dreaming of the dress I would wear down the aisle when I married the guy who I thought was the most perfect guy in school (Sean Jordan) and the color baby booties I would be knitting when I happily told him we were pregnant. Mind you, I never quite thought out how we would actually get pregnant. Somehow, I was supposed to miraculously just learn how to knit *and* end up with child.

I was hopelessly, helplessly, pitifully naïve.

But you know what? Back then, naïve was a good thing, particularly as it related to sex, and I was blissfully ignorant of the mechanics. I knew the consequences better than I knew how to spell my name, thanks to Bettye and Jimmy. But the how-tos? No haps.

And that was okay. Then.

Being stupid about and scared of sex was a part of learning

about it. We'd all heard and happily spread the legendary childish sex theories—you can't get pregnant the first time, a saltwater douche would stop the sperm from getting to the egg, pumping your elbows backward while you push your wanna-be breasts forward every night would increase your bra size. We asked each other if we'd "done it" yet and spread gossip about those who we just *knew* were lying. We coached one another on how to get him, and coaxed one another through the broken hearts—without a clue as to what we were talking about.

And our parents tried their best to avoid the sex lectures— went out of their way not to talk about it. Shoot, my mom taught me about my period by ordering me the Kimberly-Clark jumbo menstrual set—came with a bunch of books and every form of period pad, tampon, and panty liner under the sun. I was so excited to get that box, I didn't know what to do with myself—ripped it open like it was a Christmas present. My mom, I can imagine now, was just glad to see my questions were answered in the pages of those pamphlets and that I wasn't going to ask her about it. Anything else I needed to learn about my period, I simply revisited Judy Blume's *Are You There God? It's Me, Margaret.*

As far as I can see, it worked. The parents of the Brentwood High School class of 1986 did such a good job keeping us in the dark—or at least arranging it so that we wouldn't get caught out there in case we found the light—that only three of them became grandparents before graduation.

And nobody thought the impending parenthood of their daughters was cute.

In fact, it was shunned—not only by the school administration

and the parents, but the kids, too. It was irresponsible and reprehensible—said a lot about the kind of people they were. Sure, we
felt sorry for them, but we didn't condone it in any way. In fact, we
were all quite relieved, I think, that two of them dropped out of
school—who wanted to be around some fast-assed premature
mommies?—and that the third one didn't show her face around
the school too much.

Today, though, there's no room for naïveté. The teenagers
(and, in all-too-many cases, the preteens) know more than me, and
I'm a thirty-one-year-old married mom. They get their sex lessons—
and often, it's screwed-up but extremely racy information—from
MTV and BET, sexy prime-time television shows and movies, the
Internet, the newspapers and magazines, even the six o'clock news.
Judy Blume has been replaced by Lil' Kim and her nasty, stank,
take-it-up-the-butt lyrics, which even some six-year-olds know by
heart. There is no mystery in sex for kids, no opportunity for them
to explore innocence, let alone be innocent.

And even more disturbing is that, today, there is no stigma
about being caught out there. Little girls and boys who can barely
write their names—can barely add two plus two—are becoming
mommies and daddies, raising kids as they struggle to be kids
themselves. Nick and I recently visited my parents in Long Island
and went to a local mall there—and I was shocked by what I saw.
Almost every young teenage girl had a baby wrapped around her
waist or was pushing one in a stroller—like they were little acces-
sories to their wardrobe, or one of those new-fangled Tamagotchi
toys, except they pooped and cried for real. Clearly, nobody was
even fazed by my gape-jawed stares or incredulous whispers of,

"Lord have mercy—did you see how young that little girl with the baby was?" They simply pushed their strollers, yelled at their snot-nosed kids, and kept on getting up.

Don't get me started on the effect AIDS has had on our community and how it's devastated our youth.

And we ask ourselves, "How the hell did we get here?"

I could probably take a stab at it. At the top of my list is the inattention of parents to the changed American culture. Parents, busy with their own jobs and mates and lives to attend to, are letting their kids be raised by the television, the Internet, the radio, music videos, Jay-Z and DMX and the Ruff Riders—with absolutely no supervision by the grown-ups. Don't get me wrong; I'm a newpaper reporter by trade—a part of the ominous "media"—and I can't stand it when folks blame the media for society's ills, because there's much more to it than that. I argue, though, that the media is partly to blame, and parents, fully aware of this, should be more responsible in curbing how much of it their kids are exposed to. There's no reason, for instance, that I should be able to turn on my local radio station and hear a rap song with the curse words so ineffectively bleeped out that I know exactly when the rapper Jay-Z is saying the *F* word. There's also no excuse for that same radio station to play a song by Lil' Kim and Puffy clearly rapping sexually explicit lyrics, down to the position in which he's going to bang her and how he's going to make her breasts shake as he does it, early in the morning, when the kids are getting dressed for school.

But since it is being played—the radio station would argue that there's a market for it and they have the right to exercise their right to free speech—there's also no reason any responsible parent would allow my child to listen to it. I know that Nick's young son, Mazi, wouldn't be. I know that my parents wouldn't have allowed it. I know I wouldn't allow our daughter Mari to listen, at least not before I knew she was ready to understand and handle the information being meted out to her in those nasty songs and videos.

Parents who let their kids go to R-rated movies and listen to explicit songs and watch ridiculously nasty music videos and surf the Net unsupervised without providing context for any of the information being disseminated to their childrens' young minds are the ones who shouldn't be suprised if Junior is breaking his piggy bank open to help his girlfriend pay for an abortion. They shouldn't be surprised if Jane is sexually active at age fourteen, seeing as Foxy Brown is not only telling her how to dress sexy, but also how to exchange something so precious as her body for diamonds and expensive cars.

Newsflash: Fourteen-year-old boys can't afford diamonds and expensive cars, and fourteen-year-old girls shouldn't be wearing lingerie to school (even though, in some cases, they do—in outfits their own mamas bought them). And somebody needs to sit them down and tell them that.

Hardly anyone is.

I don't advocate shutting down the television and the radios and the computer to kids; they are going to get the information somehow, somewhere, from somebody. But parents can't let their kids risk what our parents did—information without context. Times are too dangerous, too hard—too fast for children these days for parents to stay silent and pray their kids got the message from the Kimberly-Clark books.

That means that talking to them about sex has to come *before* they're allowed to get really dumb information from their friends. That means that little girls need to know not only how they can get pregnant but what would happen if they did so at a young age—that babies aren't playthings to be slung on their hips when they go to the mall to hang out with their friends. That condomless sex means you can get AIDS, and that AIDS kills. That means that we can't depend on old Biggie Smalls songs to teach our boys how to be men, to be strong for themselves, their community, our future. That means that we have to pay attention to who their friends are and where they're going with them and what they're doing with them, even if that means Mom and Dad are checking their kids' computers to see what Internet spots they've hit or listening in on their phone conversations on occasion or just plain saying no to their demands for increased independence if they're clearly not ready for it. You wouldn't, after all, let a two-year-old run into the street. Why would you allow a fourteen-year-old to run into the public marketplace with no supervision or protection and do nothing to stop them from getting hit by the destructive images? They're no different than two-year-olds; they don't know how to handle the dangers out there, how to avoid the trouble. They think they know everything. We know they know nothing.

Parents have a moral and legal responsibility to know what's going on in their kids' lives—and it may not sound pretty to some, but if that means their rights are stomped on a bit, so be it. But your child will be alive and strong and smart and know how to deal.

When are parents going to get it?

Lord, I hope soon. Because their children—our children—are crying out for help.

So how about we as parents, aunties and uncles, friends, educators, mentors and grown-ups make the commitment to our teens? We wrote, and you just read, an entire book dedicated to getting men and women to talk to one another about sex, to give up the inhibitions and recognize that communication is the only way to improve our sexuality—and, ultimately, our lives. Perhaps we could make it better for our children by not leaving them in the dark, to encourage them to avoid all the stupid pitfalls and mistakes and lumps we've made and taken in our lives by *talking* to them. Honestly. Wisely. Prudently. Letting them know that there is nothing embarrassing about sex—that it's all at once the most beautiful and the most dangerous act two people could share. Helping them recognize that it's nothing to be toyed with. Teaching them that their bodies are precious, as is life-—both theirs and those that they risk creating if they're not careful.

This, of course, is a parent's ultimate inhibition.

But it's one that we need to get over.

Our future depends on it.

From a Brother

What's wrong with our black boys?

How many times do we scream out that lament, wringing our hands and furrowing our brows every time we turn on the evening news and there's another one dragged across the screen with his hoodie failing to cover his angry snarl and barely postpubescent face? Whatever he did, we know it was stupid and unnecessary and yet another symptom that our young men have unraveled out of control. Inevitably we start wondering about the future of our community—hell, what will happen to us when we need for these knuckleheads to be our leaders, to help us see a way through the troubles that are always ahead? We're gonna be in deep doo-doo, we think. We don't have a chance, we suspect.

We make the easy connection between the behavior of these boys as adolescents and the men that they will eventually become. But we don't seem to make the same connection between the messages these boys get as children and their resulting behavior as adolescents.

When I was a child, my mother put a poster on my wall that has always fascinated me. It was a composition called "Children Learn What They Live," written by Dorothy Law Nolte, and to my mother its words were as weighty and instructive as scripture. Nolte's point was that the way we treat our children determines what kind of adults they will become.

If a child lives with criticism, he learns to condemn.
If a child lives with hostility, he learns to fight.
If a child lives with ridicule, he learns to be shy.
If a child lives with shame, he learns to feel guilty.
If a child lives with tolerance, he learns to be patient.
If a child lives with encouragement, he learns confidence.
If a child lives with praise, he learns to appreciate.
If a child lives with fairness, he learns justice.

If a child lives with security, he learns to have faith.
If a child lives with approval, he learns to like himself.
If a child lives with acceptance and friendship, he learns to find
love in the world.

To my young mind, this composition was telling me that what happened to me at that time, the way the adults in my life behaved, would have some impact on me twenty years down the line. It was powerful and scary knowledge and I never forgot it, particularly when I had kids of my own.

When our little boys cry, though decades of conventional wisdom have told us not to, we still hit them with the "boys don't cry" line, particularly after they pass seven or eight. If we don't come right out and say it to them in those words, we still send them the message loud and clear as a bell. Then they grow up to be closed-off and emotionally distant young men who find all the wrong outlets for their rage and pain, and we wonder what's wrong with them. How did they become such monsters?

When our little boys play sports—and what little boys don't?—we push them into aggression, into making the tackle harder, into knocking over the defender, pushing the catcher out of the way. We push them into violence. Violence becomes their only way of grappling with obstacles. Then we pretend not to understand how they got that way. How did they become such monsters?

And when it comes to the opposite sex, mothers and sisters and aunts start fretting when their adolescent boy spends too much time with the same girl. "Why don't you go out with some other girls?" they ask, implying that monogamy is somehow bad. And don't let the girl be beneath their standards—in other words, not cute enough. They'll practically shove the boy in the direction of the cute little girl down the street to get him away from that nappy-headed girl around the corner. "Boys need to be adventurous, to have a lot of different experiences," they'll say. And, of course, what they're really doing is contributing to the early education of a future playa. Twenty years later they're all wondering why Tarik is unmarried and still trying to screw anything in panties.

My good friend Kathy Barrett Carter, who along with her hus-band, Bruce, is doing a masterful job in raising two handsome, respectful, and intelligent teenage boys, said it is a constant strug-gle to get her boys to understand that just because a girl is making herself available doesn't mean she's someone they should want to be with.

"I try to get them to recognize it's not a trophy or an accom-plishment to run around having unbridled sex with anybody and everybody," Kathy said.

But Kathy is fighting against a tidal wave of peer and societal pressure that tells boys exactly the opposite: Go out there and col-lect the trophies.

In his funny and insightful book *Reaching Up for Manhood: Transforming the Lives of Boys in America,* influential child advo-cate Geoffrey Canada states that the major difference between the sexual behavior of boys when he was growing up in the '60s and boys now is the behavior of girls.

"I wanted sex at twelve and thirteen, but the closest I came to it was slow dancing under a red light," Canada wrote. "If back at the age of twelve or thirteen we had known girls who were willing, I know what would have happened: sex, lots of it and all the time.

The reason more of us didn't become teen parents had little to do with values about family and marriage. We simply didn't know a lot about sex and couldn't find willing partners. . . . We have created a culture for boys that on one hand makes it too easy for them to become fathers and, on the other hand, teaches them nothing about what fatherhood means."

This is not to place the entire blame for the unfortunate behaviors of our young people on the girls. Surely if boys were taught to be more respectful of girls, to value them as more than sexual objects, they would care just as much about that girl's future as they do their own—in fact, not enough of them care even about their own futures—and be less concerned about pulling her into a room somewhere and having unprotected sex. But somebody has to talk to those boys about girls, about sex, about manhood. How many of us have those sorts of conversations with our young men?

Boys who have high expectations for themselves take the kind of precautions that keep them out of trouble. When I became sexually active, I knew the worst thing that could happen was my having to walk into my house and tell my parents that I got some girl pregnant. We all had big plans for me; they continued to inform me of this since the morning my mother helped me get dressed for my first day of kindergarten and, as she tied my shoes, told me that I had to do well in school so that one day I could go to Harvard. (I did even better: I went to Yale.) But with those words rattling around in my brain, even the distraction of a sweet young thang stretched out before me on a bed wasn't enough to make me forget the proper precautions, to endanger my future—not to mention the girl's future—by having unprotected sex. I had big plans.

Any adult can do this job of boosting expectations. It doesn't have to be a parent or a teacher. We all know boys in our lives who have potential; how much effort would it take to let them in on the secret, to let them know we expect great things from them? It doesn't require much effort at all. You work in an office building? Bring that boy into the office with you one day, let him see how things there work, show him a job or two for which he might be ideally suited. You put on a white lab coat every day and look through a microscope? You ever think about how interesting that view might be to the smart but aimless kid down the street?

I know we have that annual event called Take Our Daughters to Work Day. It's a wonderful idea, but let's not stop there. Our boys need to go to work too. They need it real bad. And we all need to get to work with our boys. Let's start when they're young. When they're still listening. Before they go into knucklehead mode.

If you've enjoyed Denene and Nick's sizzling tips for heating it up in the bedroom, you'll also love their first joint venture on loving in the '90s, *What Brothers Think, What Sistahs Know: The Real Deal on Love and Relationships,* available from Quill/William Morrow (ISBN 0-688-16498-6).

Yoo-hoo! Over Here: How Do We Get Your Attention?

From a Sistah

Can't count how many times I've been to a party with a bunch of beautiful sistahs, dip from head to toe, smelling good, sweet as sweet potato pie and ready to tear up the rug and expecting to tuck a few cuties' numbers into their purses by the end of the night—and they end up leaving dejected, having spent a full two hours buying themselves their own drinks and dancing in a circle with their girlfriends.

The cuties are there—dressed to kill and sipping their Henny, standing up against the wall next to their boys, simultaneously doing the two-step and surveying the room. But they don't move from that spot—unless it's to get a refill on that Courvoisier. They don't dance with anyone, except the wall and the one weave-and-leather-wearing-big-booty-spiked-heel woman in the room who looks like she's a little hot in the ass. And they hardly strike up a conversation with anyone other than their boys.

And in the meantime, we sistahs are left to feel like the wicked stepsister at the ball—unattractive, out of shape, just plain unworthy.

We thought we'd done everything we were supposed to do to get a guy interested in us. We made sure we looked cute that night. Threw a casual glance over at Mr. Two-Step—might have even tossed the booty in his direction.

Alas, no play.

No forseeable action.

Forced to go home feeling woefully inadequate—like we don't have what it takes to snag a good one.

It's a harrowing experience.

Ditto for the cute brother on the subway who sees us every morning at the same exact time at the same exact place, but ignores our behinds every single solitary day—and the cute guy at the video store, grocery store, mall, hell, anywhere we go where there are fine guys to whom we might be inclined to give some play.

Now maybe it's us—and we're sure you'll correct us if we're wrong—but it doesn't seem like brothers are into that old-fashioned way of meeting a sistah—the one where he sees a woman and, like, talks to her. Offers to buy her a glass of wine. Asks her out on a date.

It's almost as if we don't exist.

What do we have to do to attract your attention and get you to approach us?

From a Brother

Hold up; wait a minute. You're kidding, right? Because that scenario you've painted doesn't exist in any world I've inhabited. Where are these pretty, put-together sistahs just waiting to give all these brothers some play? This is surely a figment of your vivid imagination, right?

Let me give you this scenario as a reality check: We're leaning against the wall in the club with our boys, checking out all the cuties gathered in tight little circles with their girlfriends. We assume these women are at a DANCE club to DANCE. I don't think that's an outrageous assumption to make. We were excited and anxious when we got there because there were so many beautiful women in the house. We survey the scene carefully, trying to pick out the right one to approach. This is a dangerous, careful science. Make a mistake and our experiment blows up in our face, right there in front of the whole club. We are looking for a sign from anything with breasts. She must be with a group of three women or less so that our embarrassment will be kept to a minimum if we get dissed. She must look warm and fairly happy about life. This means that at some point we see a smile cross her lips. She must have hit the dance floor at some point during the course of the evening. If she has thrown a glance in our direction, all the better—but this one isn't entirely necessary (maybe she just can't see us from where she's sitting). We take about two hundred deep breaths, we maybe do a quick shot of Jack to boost our confidence, then we march across that interminable stretch of dance floor separating us from her table, we present ourselves in front of her and we let the magic words slide from our lips: "Would you like to dance?"

Invariably what we get in these situations is a very quick and decisive, "No, not now." That, of course, is the same as, "Hell no, Negro, now get out my way!" Though we try not to make it appear so, we are shattered. We walk back to our spot against the wall. Our boy, if he's truly our boy, offers a few mumbled curses in our behalf thrown in her direction. Maybe we get the nerve to try this one or two more times, but after awhile, thoroughly defeated and confused, we give up. In the bathroom, we stare at ourselves in the mirror and wonder what's wrong. Does our breath stink? Is there a large booger in our nose? Is it the color of the suit? (Maybe she doesn't like purple.) The haircut?

This happens all the time. It happens so often that we really don't understand what you're talking about when you complain about men not asking you to dance. It is truly a case of the genders looking at the same issue from perspectives as far apart as Mississippi and the motherland. Recently I was at a club with my wife, my sister Angelou and a group of her female friends who all happen to be single. The single women occasionally all danced together in a circle, looking like they were enjoying themselves. But then they'd sit down and look around the club, waiting—or so I thought. Then a man approached one of the women and asked her to dance. Immediately, she said, "No." Just like that. Wouldn't you know it— the next day this woman was complaining about not meeting any men at the club. Typical.

And forget about the subway, the grocery store or the video store—no way in hell you're giving us play in these locations. Come now—how many times have you really been willing to give some stranger play on the subway? Yeah, you might give him a smile if he's exceptionally good-looking; you might even let him talk to you. But are you really going to give this stranger a phone number or the necessary information to allow him to find you once you step off the train? I think not. I think sistahs step out the door with that

Hannibal Lecter mask on, and it takes rare and exceptional circumstances for the average brother to pry it off.

You wonder why the sistah with the weave, big booty and the spiked heels is getting all the dances and all the play? Well, for one, if she has a big booty and she's out there on the dance floor twirling it around for every brother to see, we're probably going to be lining up to get our chance to bask in its glorious rays. As for the weave, most brothers tend to care about or notice these hair issues much less than the sistahs do. If this sistah looks like she's having a good time and she's likely to dance with us, we're certainly going to give her a shot—particularly if the booty's talking to us. You're all going to look at her attributes and her clothes and figure we're shallow and superficial for going after her.

But what you all conveniently ignore is her attitude.

The sistah is enjoying herself; *she looks like fun.* This is what the brothers came to the club looking for: FUN. So we're going to be drawn to this sistah like flies on . . . well, you know.

Why do you all get dolled up and travel en masse with your girls to the dance club if you don't want to dance? What—or, more specifically, who—are you waiting for? Surely you know Denzel doesn't hit the clubs anymore.

From a Sistah

Ha-ha—very funny. Yes, we like to get our little grooves on as much as guys do on the dance floor—we'll whip off our heels and cut a rug into shreds if you give us a minute. And if a cheap Denzel knockoff asks us to dance, watch out! We're ready to get that soul clap going and sing right along with Frankie Beverly when he gets to that "Before I let you goooo, oooh-oh ooooh. Oh, I will never never never never never never never never never let you go before I go" in *"Before I Let You Go."* But *only if he looks like he's not going to give us any static.*

That's right. Static.

Y'all sistahs know what I'm talking about. It's the static that comes when Denzel Fake-ington decides that just because we told him we would dance with him it gave him the right to feel up every moving body part on our frame that his two hands can reach.

That's right: A sistah who says "yes" to a brother and takes his hand as he leads her onto the dance floor knows that a good 80 percent of the time, she better step to the dance floor prepared to pull some boxing gloves out of her bra and take on the brute strength of Mike Tyson if all she wants to do is dance.

You brothers know who you are.

We watch you work the room, going from sistah to sistah until one poor fool gets caught moving too much on a good song and you push up in just the precise second she was *really* feeling the beat and she said, "Sure, I'll dance with you." And as soon as girlfriend gets out of the two-step, dips, turns and tosses you a little booty? Oh my God, you lose your mind, throw your hands in the air and zero in for the kill—groin to booty, gyrating and twisting and sweating and stuff all over her good suit. Had you two been naked, she'd have left the floor eight weeks pregnant.

It's embarrassing as hell—you acting like a fool, connected to her backside. She tries to push you off, but you act like that's just part of her dance routine—until another song comes on and she runs terrified from the dance floor, eyes darting around the room to see just who all saw her getting felt up like a two-dollar ho in front of the entire nightclub. And he has the nerve—no, the outright audacity—to ask her for the digits as she dashes.

And trust me, every woman in the joint's done peeped it—including the thirty other ladies who refused your hand before you got to her.

Now, do you really think I'm going out like that? *Hell no!*

We sistahs would rather dance with our girls than get caught boogeying with some guy who's going to think that our two-step is his license to rub his little thing all over us.

See, when we go to the club, we do want to dance—we do want to have a good time. But we want to be respected, too. We want the man to be a gentleman—to ask us politely if we would like to dance, to keep a respectful distance from us while we're on the dance floor and to say "thank you" after it's over—without pressuring us into standing over by the bar and telling him our life story as he "please baby, please baby, please baby, baby, pleases" his way through his request for the digits, or, worse yet, an after-the-club date.

We just want to dance—and, perhaps, assess the chemistry from a healthy distance.

If we hit it off, then cool—we'll talk to you. And it might actually result in the exchanging of phone numbers. But if we just want an innocent dance—one with no strings (or groins) attached, respect that. Then maybe we'll be more inclined to accept that dance card.

Speaking of dance cards: What would you think if we asked you for a dance—or, better yet, out on a date—after we showed you love up in the club?

From a Brother

First, we'd fall to the floor and kiss your feet—granted they looked well-scrubbed and relatively corn-free. Then we'd stand up, give you a gracious bow in honor of your wisdom and foresight, and say, "Hell yeah, I'll go out with you!"

These are the kinds of questions that brothers don't understand. Why would we have a problem with a woman asking us out on a date, as long as we were available and interested? It relieves us of the pressure and possibility of getting dissed.

When I was in elementary school, it was common practice for girls to write those little notes to boys they liked, asking the boys to check the "yes" or "no" box to indicate whether they liked the note-writer in return. Sometimes the note even got passed to the object of the girl's affections through another intermediary, a friend of the boy. But the point was that it eventually got there, it announced the girl's intentions and feelings, and it made the boy a happy little dude for the rest of that day and probably that week. (Of course, little boys being little boys, he may not have always had the proper response. He might've decided that he didn't want to be so transparent about his answer, so he might've started a fight with her or thrown her in the mud first to camouflage his extreme pleasure.)

So, what happened to all that elementary schoolgirl aggression? What killed it over the years? Was it this notion that men liked to be the aggressors, the pursuers—a notion furthered by women such as those who wrote that book *The Rules*?

I'm here to announce that although some men may tell you

they like to be the aggressors, there's likely not a man in the world who isn't thrilled by the idea of a woman making the first move. (Unless your name happens to be Michael Jordan or Wesley Snipes, both of whom probably get nauseated by all the luscious beauties throwing themselves at them. Tough life.)

We can't repeat enough that we're just as frightened by getting dissed in a club as you're all frustrated because not enough of us ask you to dance. There's a major problem here, a logjam that won't be broken unless somebody is bold enough to make the first move. I wish more men could toss their feelings and their egos to the side and approach every woman in the club for a dance. But you know how that would look. That brother would soon become a clubwide joke as the crowd witnessed the rejections start to pile up. In the absence of bigger male *cojones,* we need some help from the females. More aggression on your part would go far in breaking the logjam. Who knows—some of y'all might even find husbands.

But I ask of you, please, be realistic. If you know you're no Halle Berry, if you have more in common with bassett hound than Angela Bassett, don't march up to the best-looking brother in the club and expect him to be thrilled by your invitation. If he's a nice guy, he might agree to dance with you, but he's not going to be wild about spending the rest of the evening with you at his side, chasing away all the cuties. This is shallow and evil, you say? (See Chapter 3 on the importance of appearance.) I offer in evidence Exhibit A: The devastating ugliness that ensues when the pudgy brother with the bad teeth and nonexistent rap saunters up to Fly Girl, interrupting her love affair with her vanity mirror, and asks her to join him on the dance floor. Are onlookers more likely to say Fly Girl was shallow, or to ask themselves what in the world could Brotherman have been thinking?

If you use this book to initiate dialogue or just to make your partner laugh, we'd love to hear about it. Write to us at

Chilmill Publishing Inc.
P.O. box 747
South Orange, New Jersey 07079
or E-mail us at our website, www.celebrateblacklove.com